Goddesses Don't Eat Green Bananas
by Lesley Daley

For Brown.

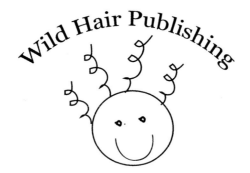

1st. Edition 2005
Copyright @ 2005 by: Wild Hair Publishing

Printed in Ventura, California

ISBN: 090765991.txt

VISIT WEBSITE: goddessbook.com

Production Consultant: 451 Media | www.fourfiftyone.com

Goddesses Don't Buy Green Bananas!

When imagining a Goddess what comes to mind? A gorgeous female with fantastic presence, striking features and a famous body? One might more insightfully define a Goddess as an ultimate achiever, honored for her meaning as a woman and her contributions to humanity. A true Goddess is surely a woman of strength, power and grace. It may further be understood by those who know her well that she is also a mistress of patience and endurance, too hard-won and little-known keys to success. Such a woman is filled with inner beauty, elegance, and harmony. I now know many, and wish to share them all with you. The Goddesses in this book are superwomen, who fight and keep at bay any threat encountered, including cancer.

Goddesses don't dwell on uncertainty when life deconstructs around them. Goddesses resist weakness; they love and they embrace every ounce and sign of life. Stirring and spreading the life force keeps Goddesses very busy. They are marvelously busy unto themselves, but also in high demand. Goddesses don't have time to stop and rest. They are the life force, and because of this they never really die.

Goddesses don't have time to wait around for green bananas to ripen!

What would you do if somebody you loved were diagnosed with a horrible disease? At 35 years old you think you are invincible from illness, let alone a deadly one. The Friday morning that my husband was diagnosed with cancer, my sheltered reality was forever altered. He insisted that he was not going to die. It was now up to me to maintain confidence and help us both through a new and dreadful course. But how?

I became obsessed with information on cancer. I read every book I could find. I went on the Internet and found myself lost in a maze of medical terminology. One website led to another. Each day of research became a full-time job. I had files bulging with information, but most were useless. I required more and more. When I exhausted all the websites, I found myself addicted to medical racks in bookstores. I was driven to absorb prodigious amounts of information and did not want a single bit of data to get past me.

I discovered that most chemotherapy makes your hair fall out. Therefore, I bought my husband 15 different hats. I read about the miracles of green tea. I had my husband drinking three cups a day. I was very pleased to find that it was contained in many other foods; I think his skin gradually turned a pale shade of emerald.

I learned that radiation could cause sterility, and thus convinced my husband that we would need to bank his sperm. While we were not even planning to have children, even the thought of not being entitled was threatening. I read about Lance Armstrong and his super-human bout with cancer and winning *The Tour de France*. I read about Gilda Radner and while hers was a wonderful story, the ending was so sad.

Nowhere did I read, "You and your husband will endure this moment in time."

I needed to be strong and confident for my husband, and he needed to lean on me. Where was I going to get the strength? I felt isolated. Nobody I knew had experienced this particular agony. I needed a role model and an ally. Then, I remembered an extraordinary woman that I had the good fortune to meet a year before my husband's diagnosis. As a professional photographer, I had the opportunity to create a black and white portrait of this middle-aged mom and her daughter. Their relationship and chemistry was amazing. During the photo shoot, Gayle, the mom, who had been in remission for one year, shared her experience with breast cancer. She looked dazzling and healthy in astounding contrast to what we all envision of a woman who just had a mastectomy and a bone marrow transplant. Gayle had started swimming and had the robust upper body to prove it. It was meeting her that made me know I needed to take advantage of the expressions of photography. I draped Gayle's muscular shoulders with a silky flowered material and wrote in script with a black marker above her heart, the word, "*SURVIVOR.*"

When Gayle received the finished "survivor" photograph, she requested several copies to give out and pass around. She said the message was evident; she was strong and brave. She gave a picture to the doctor who had saved her life. She gave one to her best friend who had held her hand through all the treatments. She gave one to each of her children. She even framed one for her living room fireplace mantel, so that she is constantly reminded that she did survive and did so powerfully and courageously. Thanks to Gayle, I realized that I could express emotion through my photographic portraits.

The project evolved. This book set forth and created itself. I would photograph women who were currently undergoing cancer treatment or were recently in remission.

The first lovely lady I photographed with the book in mind was Clarice, a 70 year old living with Non-Hodgkin's Lymphoma. My husband and I met her at the Blood-Cancer Support Group. She always sat across from us, holding her husband's hand. They had been married 50 years. Creating her portrait was simple and the interview was effortless. It was the final image that revealed her story; no words were necessary. Clarice's husband, Sonny, sat with her; his face buried in her neck, his eyes were closed. Clarice faced the camera with a resolute smile that showed off her tranquility. Love was their guide; love helped them through the fear. It was all they needed. I captured this sentiment.

The word got out in the cancer community; women started to contact me. They had stories to share. At first their fearless, uncensored tales offered me a distraction from "my" problem. I discovered genuine heroism. My fears slowly transformed into hope. These women I worked with were forced to take a detour in their lives because of cancer.
Each one was just too young, too much in love or had too much work to do. There is not a right time to get cancer. It takes away too much; it does not care who you are. Cancer shows no respect for age, beauty, wealth or fame.

I photographed and wrote the stories of triumph, conviction, power, bravery, strength and the importance of 37+ phenomenal women whose lives were rearranged by cancer, because their stories had to be told. I have grown healthier from time spent with these women and I wrote this book so that others can feel better too by experiencing what it means to fight and work your way successfully through the craziness.

Thank you for reading this book!

Lesley

Lesley Daley

One last note---All references to time have been removed in the book. It's all about today!

Gloria's Introduction

I am honored to contribute to the introduction of this heart-felt compilation of some extraordinary photos of some extraordinary people.   As the Executive Director of the Cancer Center of Ventura County at St. John's Regional Medical Center in Oxnard, California.   I am always in awe of the people that I meet.   Many of them have become my friends. As a nurse, those who are faced with a life threatening or chronic disease have inspired me. When my father was first diagnosed with diabetes and then with lung cancer, he took action to fight.
He taught me the importance of living ever day to its fullest. As you will witness in this photo journal, my friends have great spirits that tell their stories touching many emotions.   This remarkable collection of art will have you thinking about those diagnosed with cancer in a new way.   Lesley Daley has superbly captured the beauty of these people.   Her experience with cancer began when she worked as an oncology nurse.   Even more poignant was when her husband, Jim was diagnosed with cancer. In her attempt to heal, she was able to take her photographic expertise and combine personal experience with her commentaries for a book that is a unique testament to the human spirit.   So, grab a couple of tissue; meet and experience the journey of women with cancer who have thrived.

Gloria Forgea, RN, MBA

Everybody Knows Somebody Who has Had or Has Cancer!

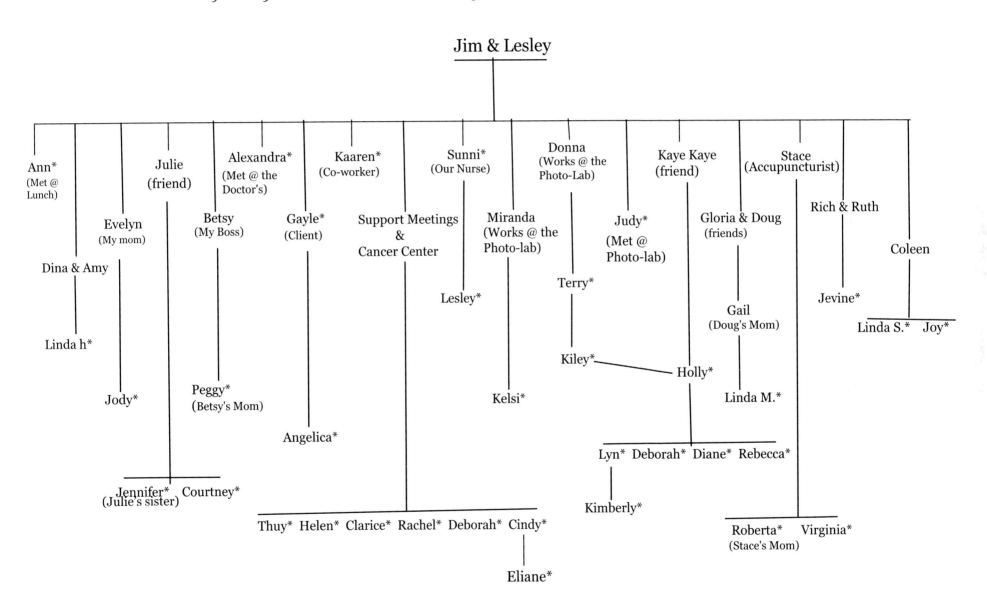

*Goddess (appear in the book)

A father's tale...

With the stirring Goddess-filled pages ahead, Lesley Daley has accomplished something highly unusual and most commendable. She has creatively and sensitively managed to humanize a subject that a few decades ago people would rather not talk about in polite society. Welcome to the 21st Century! Today, we have learned that cancer and many other devastating diseases must be constantly pushed to the media's foreground as a prereqisite to their eventual defeat. Lesley's labor of love helps us all to enthusiasically celebrate the increasingly encouraging statistical facts that many thousands DO survive and Do go on to live productive lives.

One of these plucky and genuine Goddesses is my lovely daughter who adorns the opposite page with the word *Survivor* emblazed above her steadfast heart. She was diagnosed 14 years ago, just six months before her beloved mother, Judy, succumbed to the same disease; breast cancer. Gayle has seen it all, the good days, the bad days, the little victories and rays of sunshine, but also the occasional downs, which she would not accept for one minute. (With the help of caring doctors' and a fomidable support system captained by a loving spouse and her devoted children and joined by an awesome legion of family and friends, Gayle wears her surviorship graciously). As her dad, I could be not prouder...nor more grateful.

Lesley's beacon of light herein deserves not only to be seen, but also to be studied and admired. This precious display of ultimate compassion has touched the souls of all of us who have previewed these pages. It is much too important not to reach the multitudes.

Spread the word!

Stuart F. Tower,
Father & author

Los Angeles, California
2004

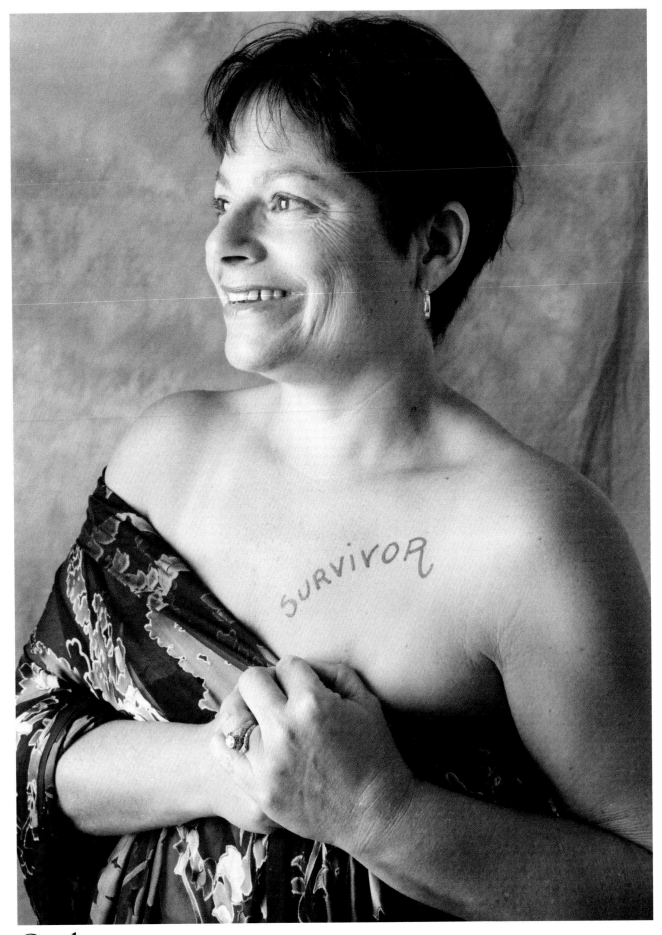

Gayle

Alexandra

Goddess of...Conviction, Appreciation of Western Medicine and Recognition of family significance.

I am 28 years old and have a 14-month old daughter. I went to the doctor for a routine visit and the doctor found a hard lump in my left breast. This surprised me because there is no history of cancer in my family. I never thought about cancer, I just assumed you had a mammogram at 30 years old. The doctor did a needle biopsy and it was normal.

The lump was taken out; even if it was not cancer, it was growing fast. Unfortunately, the tests showed that it was cancer. I had a mastecomy with 31 lymph nodes removed. Two weeks later a second tumor was found in the axially area.

I had chemotherapy; six outpatient treatments. (I went once a week every three weeks). My chemotherapy drugs were, Adriamycin, Taxol and Cytoxan. When I would see the IV, I saw it as a cure, not as a a bad thing.

I had a bad allergic reaction to Taxol; I could not breath. The doctors stopped treating me with Taxol after that happened.

During all of this, I have been depressed, panicked and scared for strength. I still work and I take dance classes. I used to be the planner type, but now I think more for the moment.

I feel lucky to be in the USA--the treatment here is better than in Columbia.

My support system is wonderful--my husband and sister are great. My baby girl is perfect. She likes to touch my head since I don't have hair, and then she touches her head, because she doesn't have hair either. Her new word is "HAT."

I am brave!

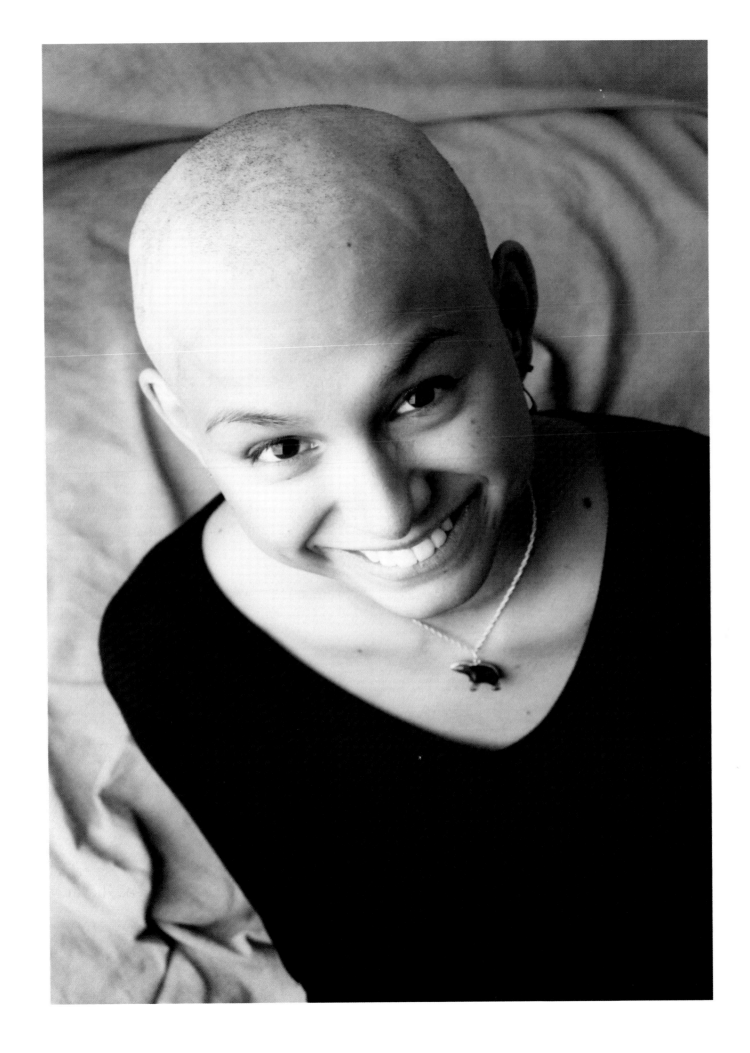

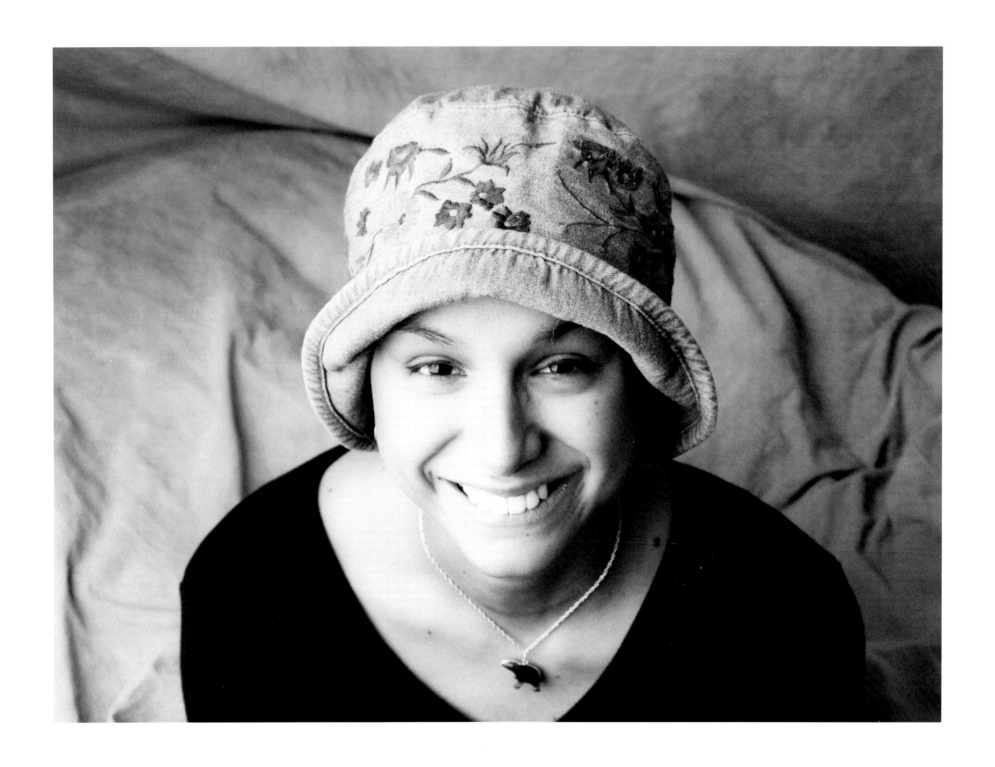

"Be faithful in small things because it is in them that your strength lies."

Mother Teresa

I am a soft-spoken and gentle person. I was born and raised in Columbia. My husband is an American. We met and fell in love while he was living in Columbia in order to master Spanish.
We have been married six and a half years and have a 14-month-old daughter named Isabella.

My sister Olga is 33 years-old and my childhood bedmate. She came to visit me in the United States three years after I moved here. During her visit, unexpectedly Olga fell in love with my husband's best friend. Then, Olga relocated to the United States to start her new life.

We are not only sisters, but inseperable best friends. We now reside in the same country once again. Olga has really helped me through all of this.

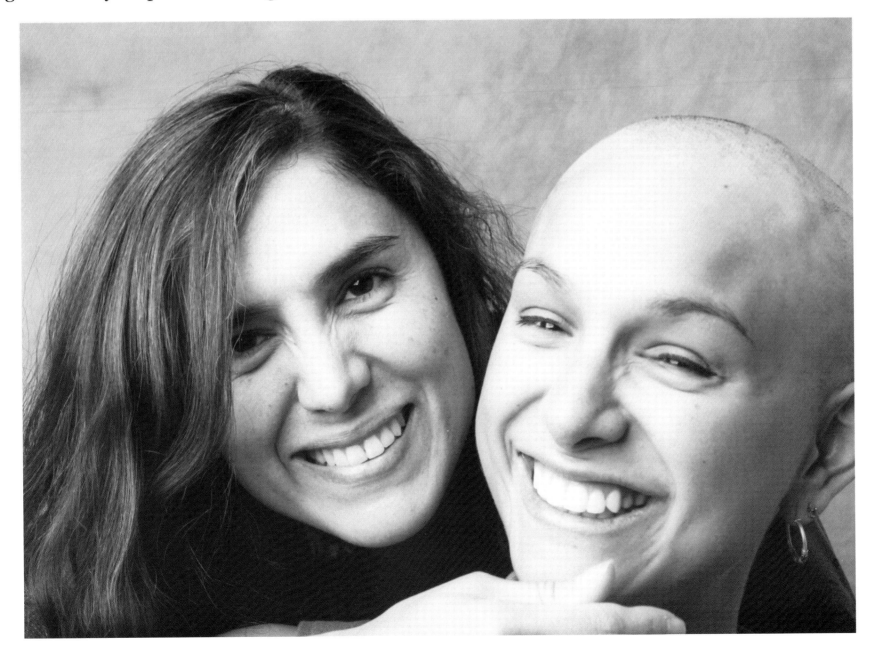

Kimberly... Goddess of Innocence, Spunk and Chocolate

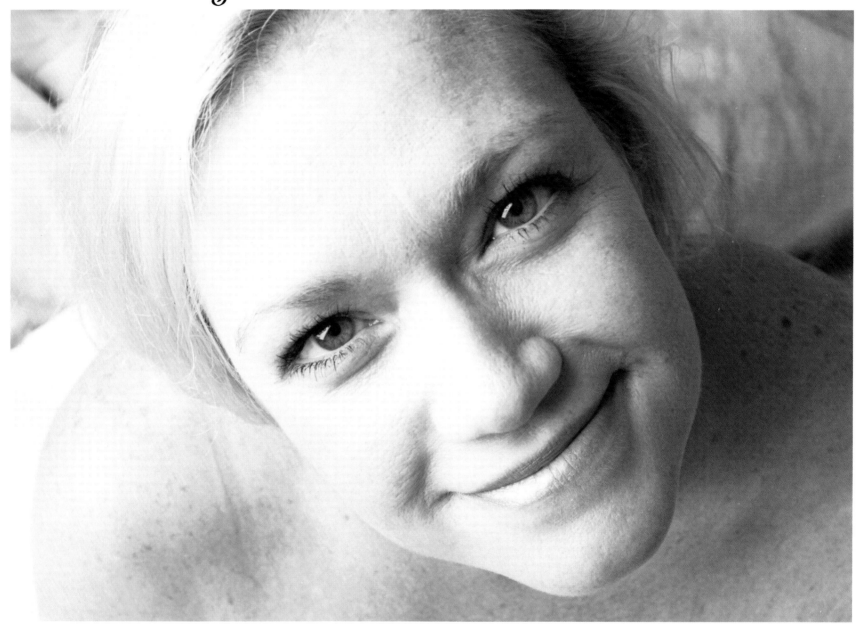

I have a long history for someone that is only 35 years old. I was raised by my grandma, Naomi Knight. She died of pancreatic cancer. I feel like she is now my guardian angel. When I was 18 years old, I was diagnosed with **Hodgkin's Lymphoma**. I had chemotherapy for one year. Then, I was diagnosed with melanoma, which was located near my underarm and breast. It was removed by surgery. A couple years later, I was diagnosed with Sjogrens syndrome. (Prounounced: SHOW-grins) This is an autoimmune disease that attacks the moisture-producing glands (such as the eyes and mouth) and causes fatigue.   Recently, I have been diagnosed with Lupus. From all of this, I have 17 surgical scars.

I cope with life by writing poetry, eating chocolate and watching MTV. I do not waste time by questioning, "Why me?' I have two sons and lots of friends.

I always keep smiling!

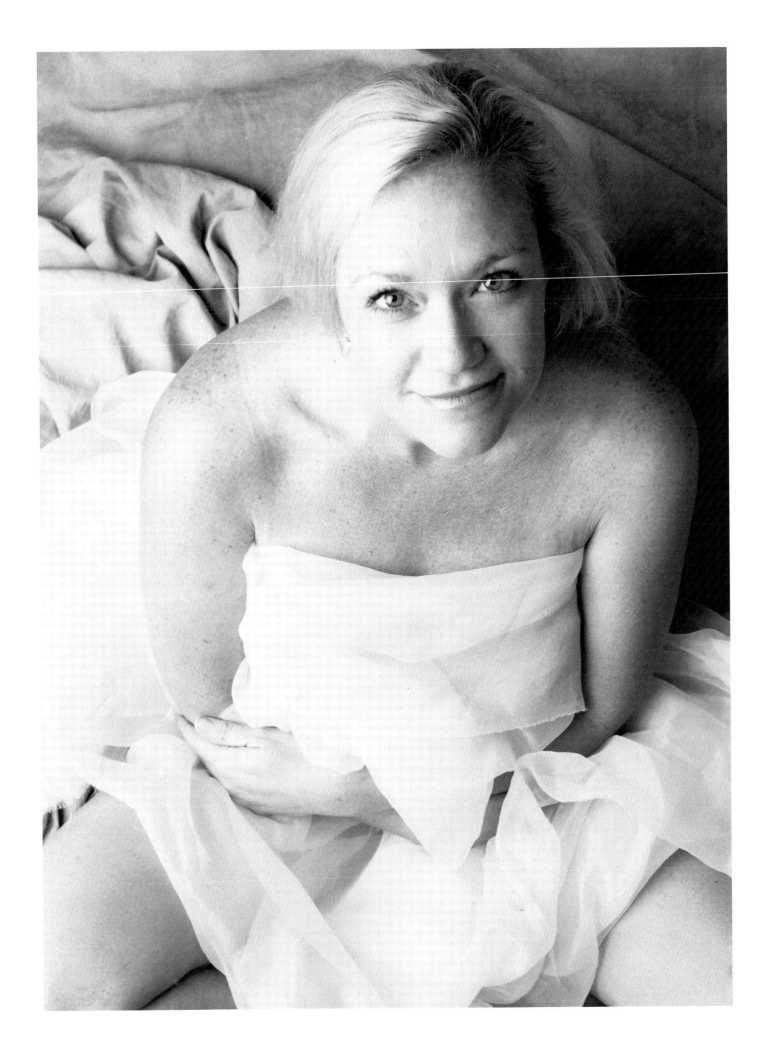

Gayle
Goddess of... Friendship and Survival

In 1990 my mother, at age 59, had end-stage breast cancer. She urged me to have a mammogram; I was only 33 years old. Luckily, I took my mother's advice. Unfortunately, the mammogram showed that I had breast cancer too. I had a right mastectomy, radiation and chemotherapy. My mother lived six months into my treatment.

Before my mom died, we had some time to support each other and endure the pains of cancer as partners. We were bald from chemotherapy, used to try on wigs together, invent different scarves to wear, and go to our radiation treatments.

I started reconstruction but I did not finish. I did not want more surgery. Being alive was the most important thing, and my husband was totally supportive of my decision.

 After I went into remission, I had a baby and I did not think this was possible. We called him our miracle baby. I nursed him with one breast.

A few years later, I noticed a lump on my neck. It was metastatic breast cancer and had spread to my lymph nodes and to my spine. To me, that meant a death sentence- this is what my mom had. This completely freaked me out.

I was treated aggressively. I had three months of chemotherapy, and two piggy-back stem-cell transplants. Prior to the transplant, the doctors took me down to death by wiping out my entire body of blood cells, so that you can start over with the transplanted cells. Anyone that is in your room has to wear a mask- you basically have no immune sytem to fight any germs.

During this time, there were two people that never left my side- my husband Michael and my best friend Julie. They took turns staying at the hospital and watching the children at home. WOW!

I love to do yoga and swim to stay in shape. I try to stay active and think positively.

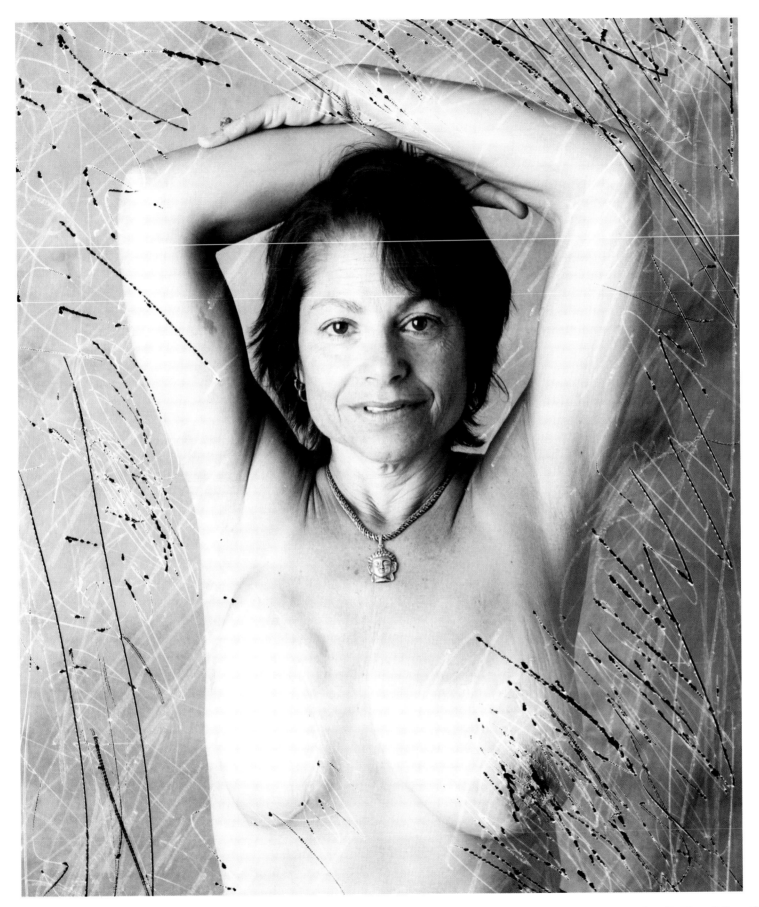

"I BREAST FED MY NEWBORN SON WITH ONE BREAST."

Gayle & Julie.... The ultimate ties of a best-friendship

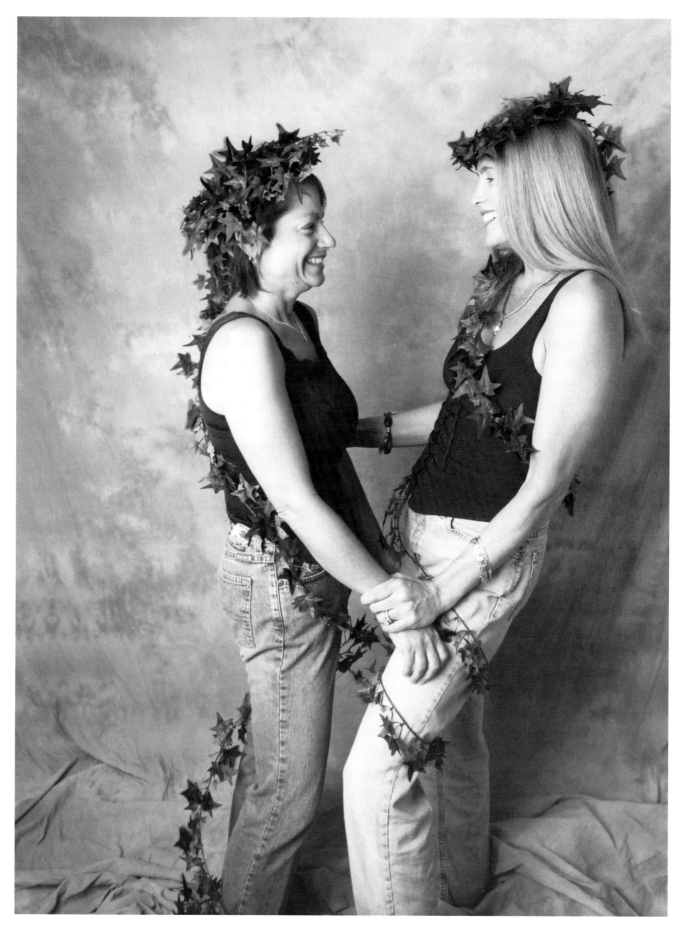

Gayle and Julie

Julie gave up one year of her life so that she could save mine!

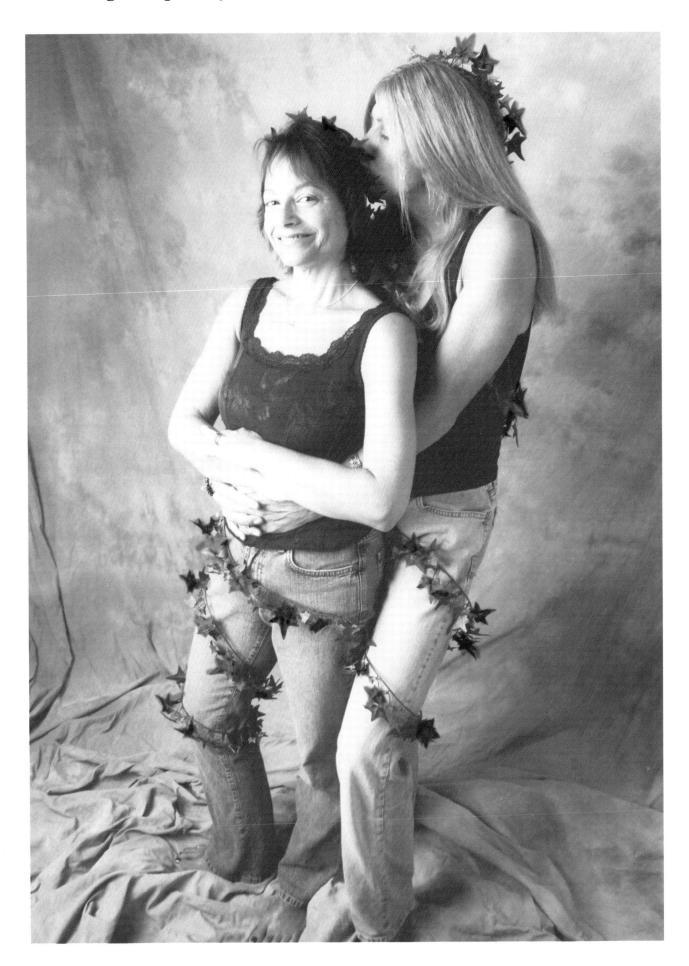

Clarice *Goddess of...* Commitment and Love

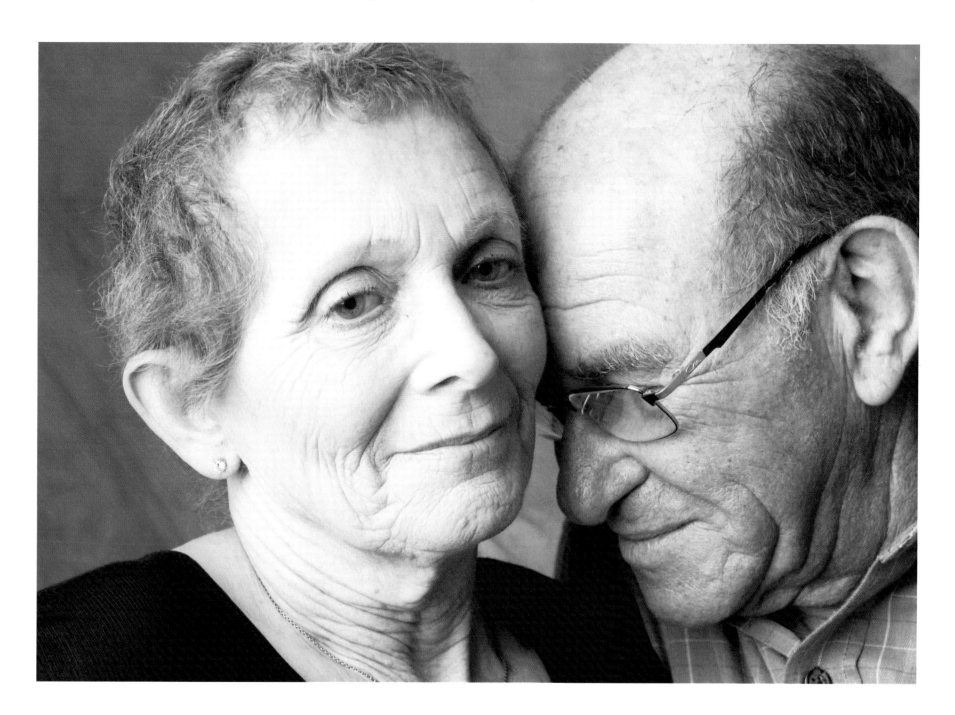

Clarice & Sonny

*We have been married 50 years...
we are still very much in love!*

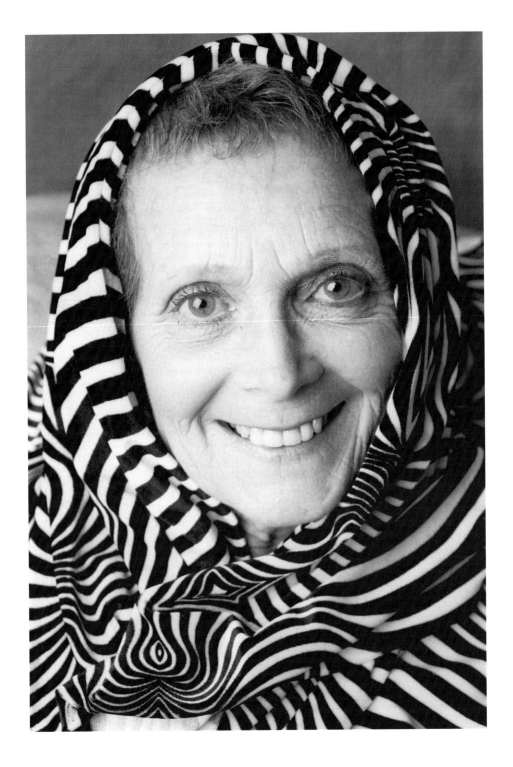

I am 70 years old. I was oringally diagnosed with both Non Hodgkin's Lymphoma and Hodgkin's Lymphoma. I was treated with Chemotherapy. I was in remission, but the cancer came back. I have been consulting with the best doctors that we can find, they are at Stanford Hospital. My husband and I go to support groups and learn as much as we can about this disease. There is a lot to learn.

I had to renew my drivers license about the same time my hair started to grow back. I had to fill out the application with personal information, such as, the color of my eyes and the color of my hair. My husband said that my new hair color was taupe. It made me laugh, because I did not think he even knew what that color was.

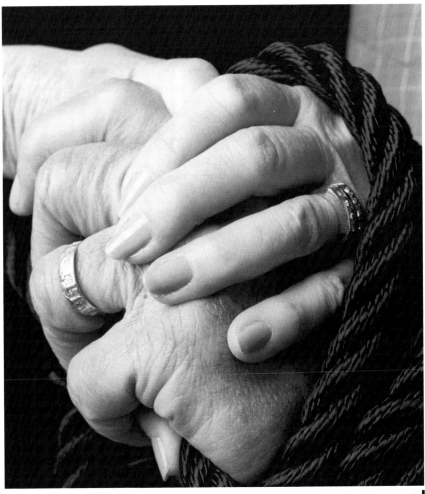

Today, I am feeling well and I am trying not to think about this too much!

Angelica

Goddess of... The Ocean and The Ability to Over Come

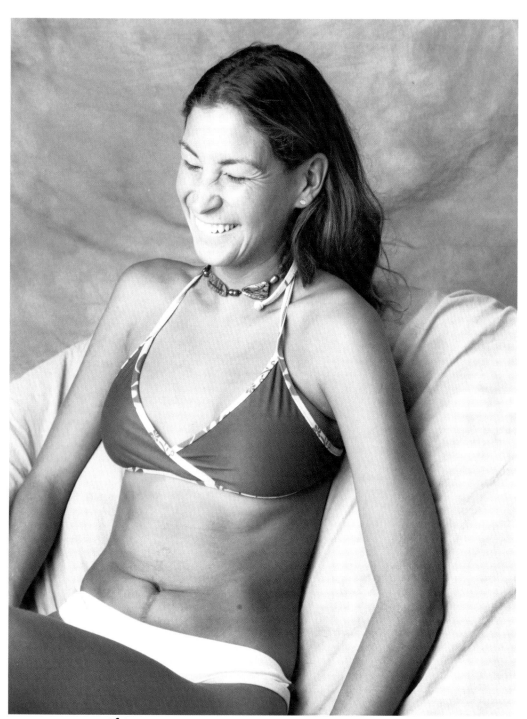

If I ever got cancer again...

I was diagnosed with ovarian cancer when I was 17 years old. It was found by a routine pap-smear. I had a second opinion with an ultra-sound. One week later I had one ovary removed. Two days later, I had a total hysterectomy.

The cancer was also in my lymph-nodes, so I had to have chemotherapy--
I had three different kinds.

I was so embarassed when I lost my hair, since I was living in a "Barbi-Doll" kind of town.

Cancer had made me face my fears. One fear was the ocean. I learned to surf.

I have also changed my lifestyle. I am a vegetarian and I like to learn about nutrition. I eat a lot of beans and grains.

I am 24 years old and newly married to Chris. He is a professional surfer. We have three dogs, two cats and four new kittens.

My husband is really cool about my infertility. He is such a positive influence and this balances me.

I am a Virgo---so I think too much.

My mom is a strong woman and she is supportive.

I would fight again!

"Today, my husband & I run a surf camp. I am living my dream"

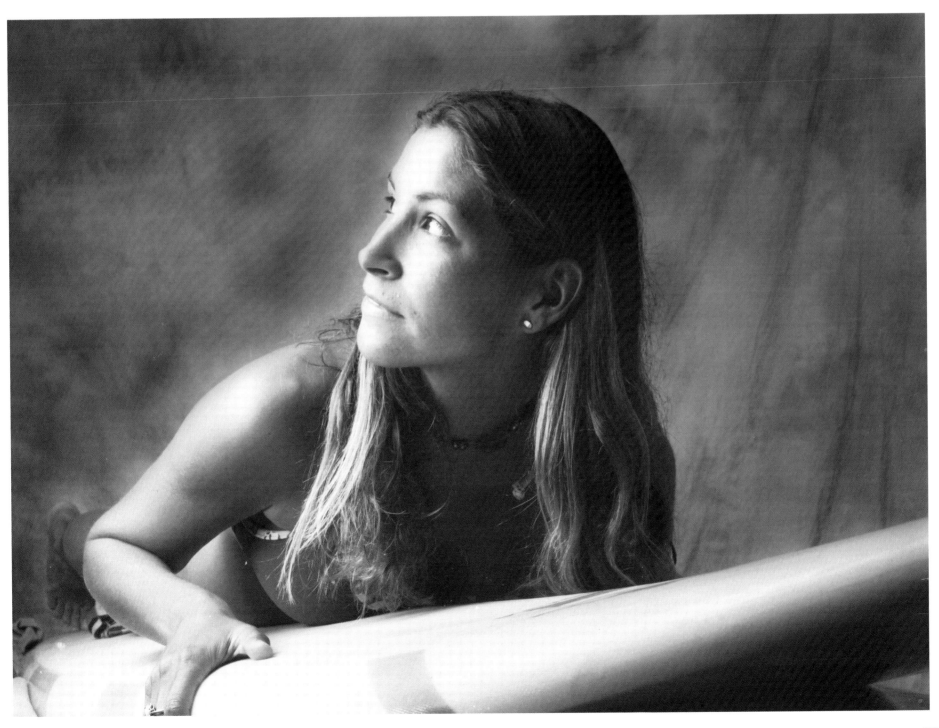

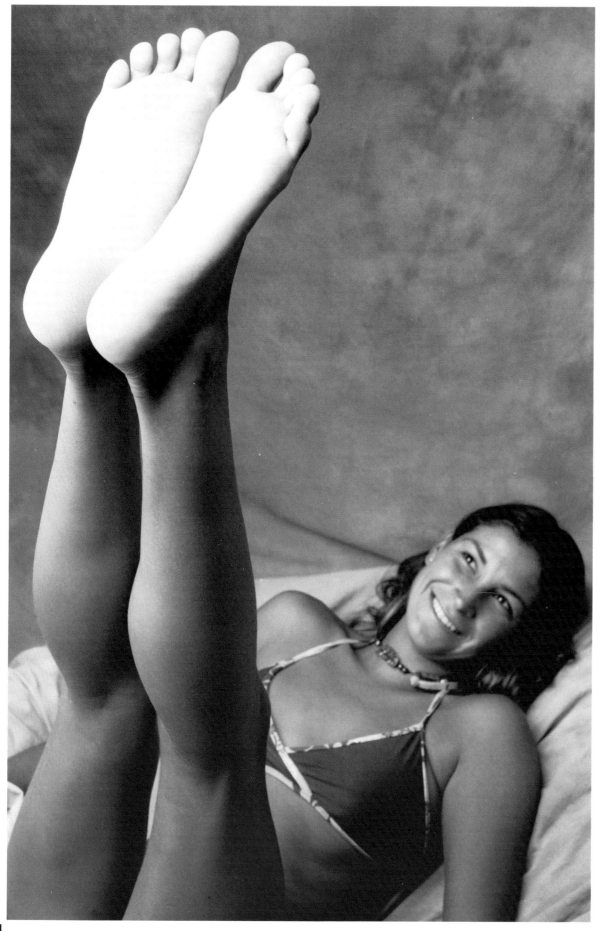

My License
plate says...

"Eat Life"

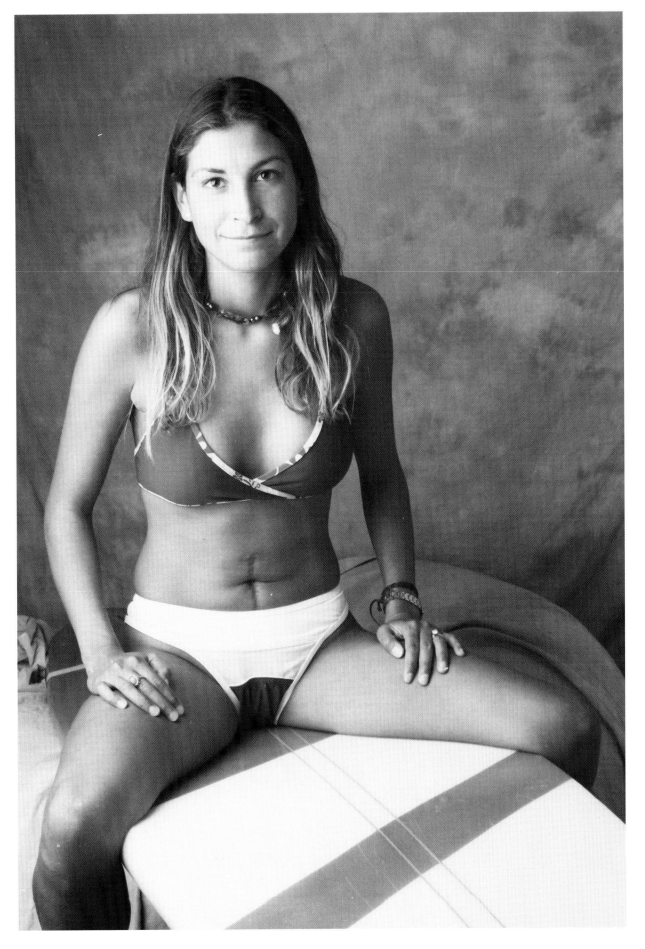

Even though I have a
surgical scar down my
entire belly...
I am still proud to wear
a two-piece bathing suit.

Lyn
Goddess of....
Passion, Partnership and A Confidant for Others!

My story is short and simple.

I had already lost a sister to breast cancer, so when I was diagnosed, I feared the same fate for myself. But angels who were not only in heaven watched over me: here on eath they surrounded me too. They gave me strength and determination and most of all...their love. I don't have to mention their names because they know who they are, but the one who stands out above the rest is my husband, Jeff!

These photographs symbolize him surrounding me with love and strength, and that's what got me through this.

It's been six years since my diagnosis: life is great!

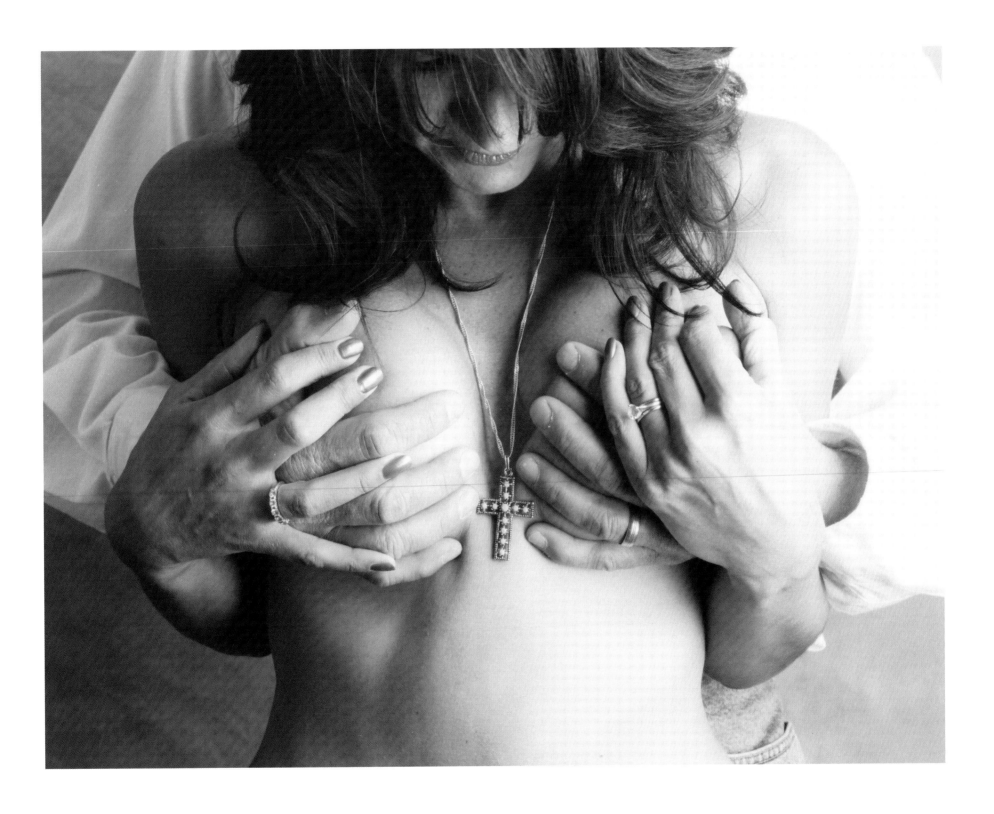

My husband is my Best Friend!

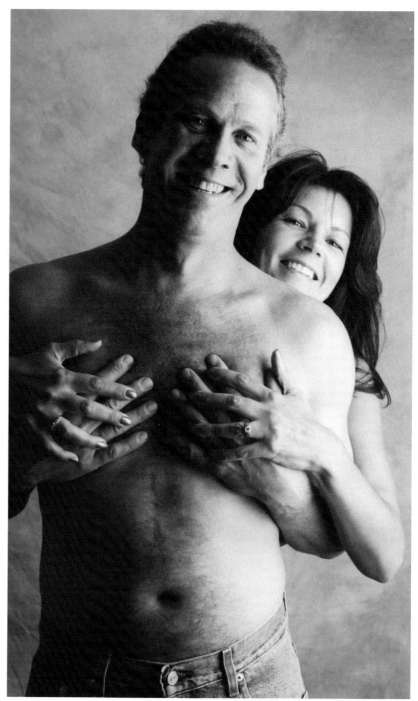

Jeff and Lyn

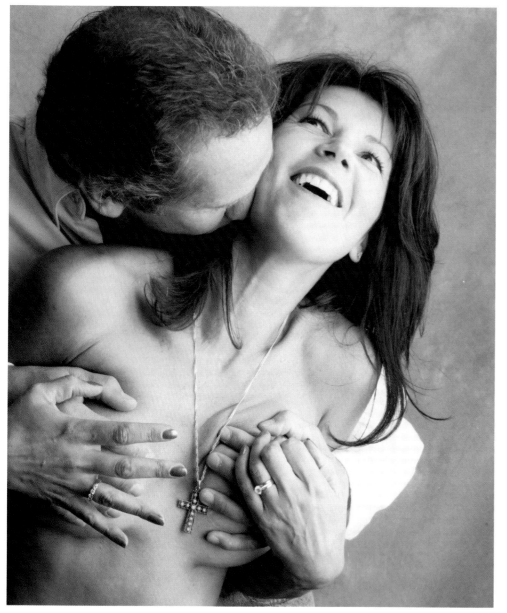

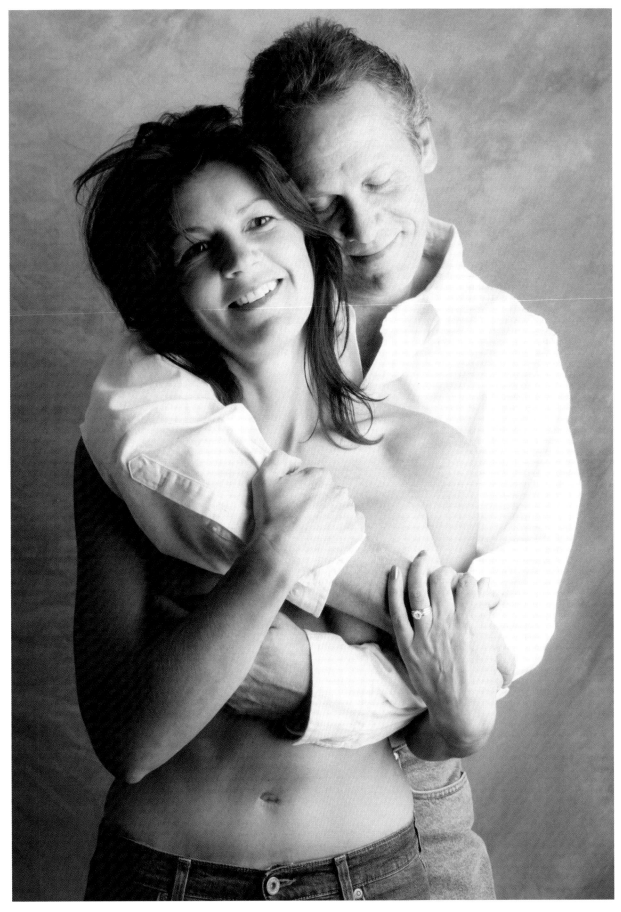

I volunteer for Reach for Recovery and hope that I can give a little strength to someone else facing this dreaded disease.

Goddess of... Affection and Craft

ANN

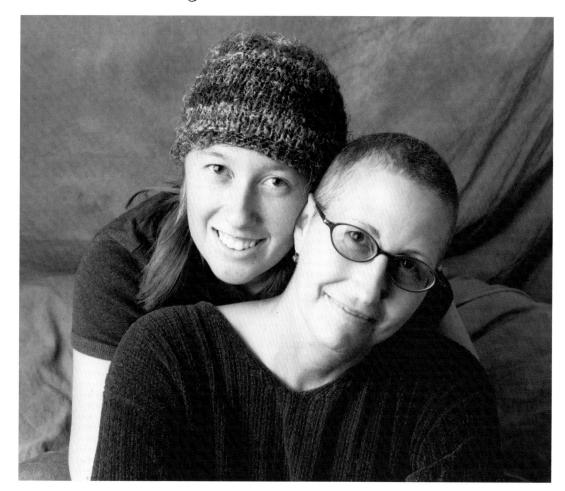

Ann & Lahti

I am 49 years old, married to Andy and we have a daughter named Lahti and a son named Dutch.
I had cancer in my left breast. Prior to my diagnoses, I had been complaining of pain for nearly
two years, I was told it was "just" a swollen duct. It turned out that I had Ductile Carcinoma.
The first lumpectomy was not clear. My second surgery was when the lymph node and surrounding
tissue were removed. (At that time the margins were clear). Then I had four rounds of chemotherapy.
I thought it would not bother me, but when they injected it into my veins I felt sad. Then, I lost my hair.
I was now offically a "Chrome Dome." The radiation was not nearly as bad as the chemotherapy.

I love being a mom---I've been one for 20 years. However, now it's time to find ANN.
I need to focus on happiness.

I love to "cane" on furniture. (Look at the seat of the rocking chair in the picture on the next page, it was
caned by Ann) I love babies and have this urge to snuggle with them. There is a volunteer job
at the community hospital where you work as an official "Cuddler" in the nursery. I cannot wait to start.

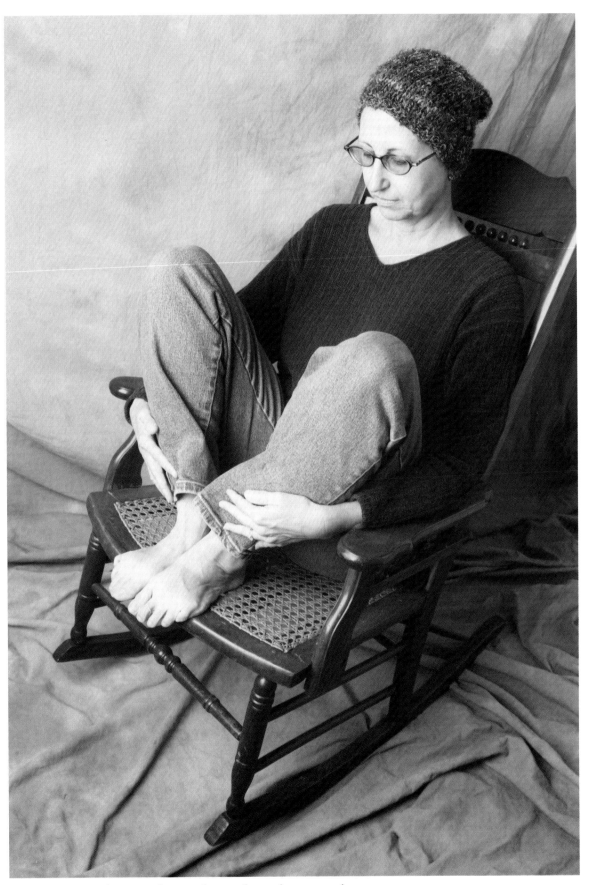

Anne sits in her rocking chair that she caned.

Peggy & Brie

(Grandmother)   (Granddaughter)

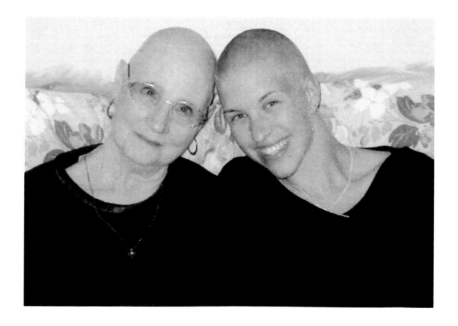

I am 70 years old and have been married 50 years. I am a strong woman who has turned more internal.

In December,I had shortness of breath and was taken to urgent care, after 18 months of tests, blood transfusions, EKG's and bone marrow biopsies, the tests finally showed that I had Multiple Myeloma—there is no cure! I thought, "how are we going to handle this?"

This cancer eats away at your bone marrow and is usually found after a bone is broken.

I entertained everyone in the hospital; I had satin pajamas.

One year later, I started chemotherapy-- five days a week for three sessions. My family was in shock. At home I received chemotherapy through a port-a-cath and wore the medication in a fanny pack. I did this for two months. Then I was told that the chemotherapy wasn't working. Big surprise!

I am taking Thalidomide. This makes me sleepy, so I take it at 9pm, right before I go to bed. I had heard about this medication through a conference where all the *biggies* [important people in the medical field] were. The medication mutates the cancer cells in the bone marrow. I have to get my prescription renewed every month through the government. Each time I call I get interrogated with such questions; age, last menstrual period, etc. --they are very strict.

When my hair fell out, my granddaughter Brie shaved her head. She did not tell anyone she was going to do this, not even her mom. We both avoided looking in the mirror when we were bald. She did it to support me, not to gain attention. Yet, her actions snowballed into a big thing. Brie started talking at churches about courage and strength. She said, "you can tell people's morals by the way they reacted."

Brie's hair grew quickly and nicely. My hair was snow-white. I got it dyed blonde.

Today, I am in partial remission—stable. I was given a two-year prognosis; it's been two and half years since I heard that. I am more frightened now that I am in remission; I am afraid that I will outlive my husband. I thought I was going to die and I worked hard preparing to face death.

My goals--to see my granddaughter graduate college
and to dance at her wedding.

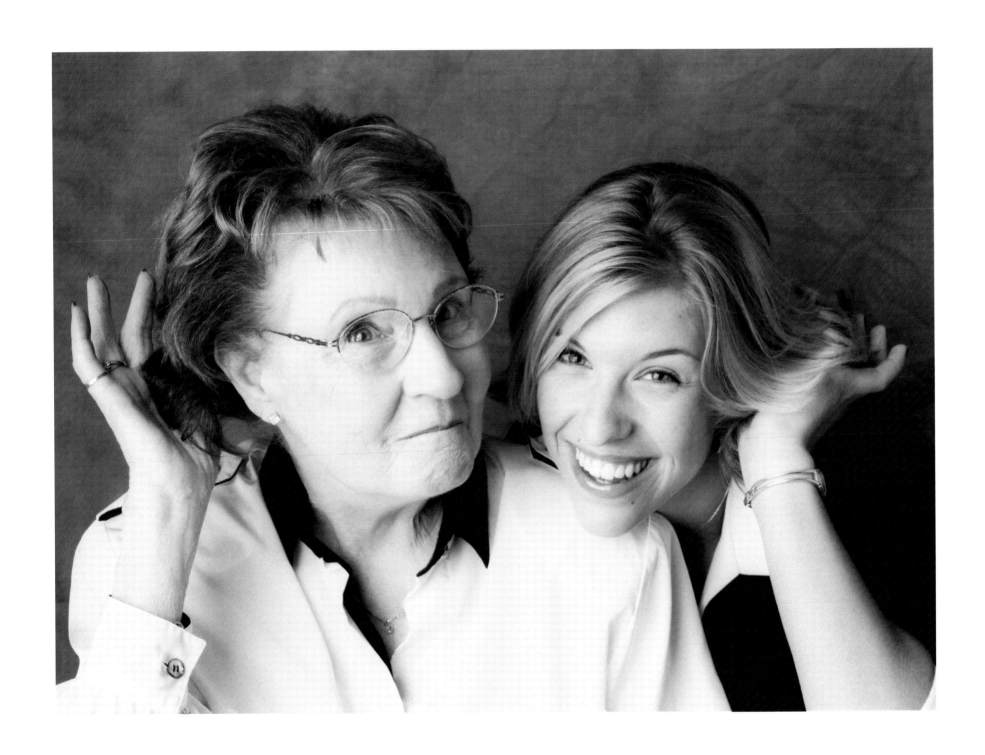

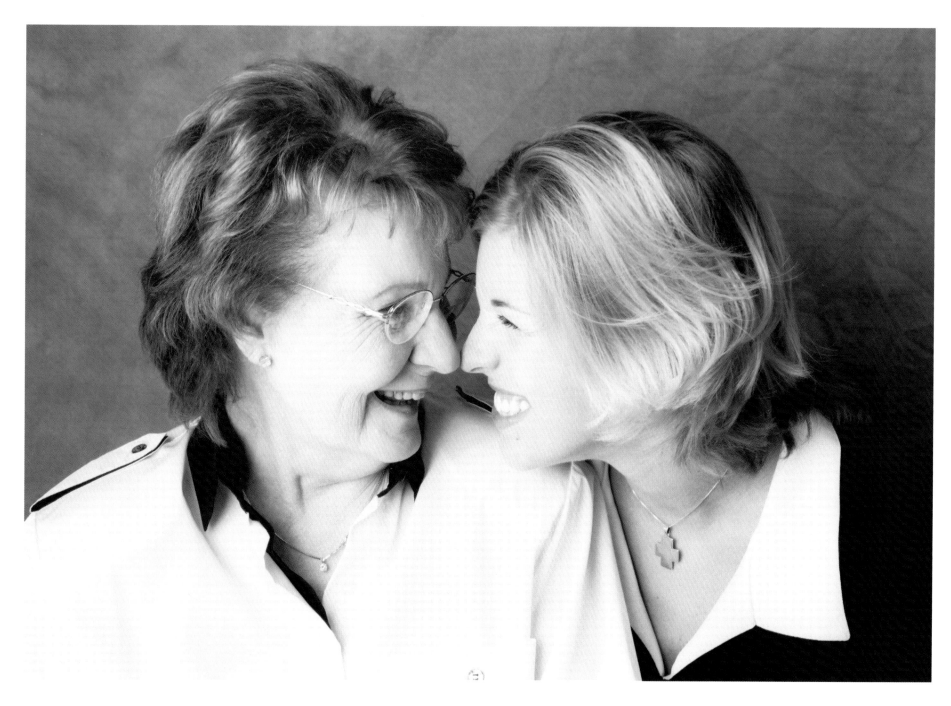

Our bond has touched lots of people.

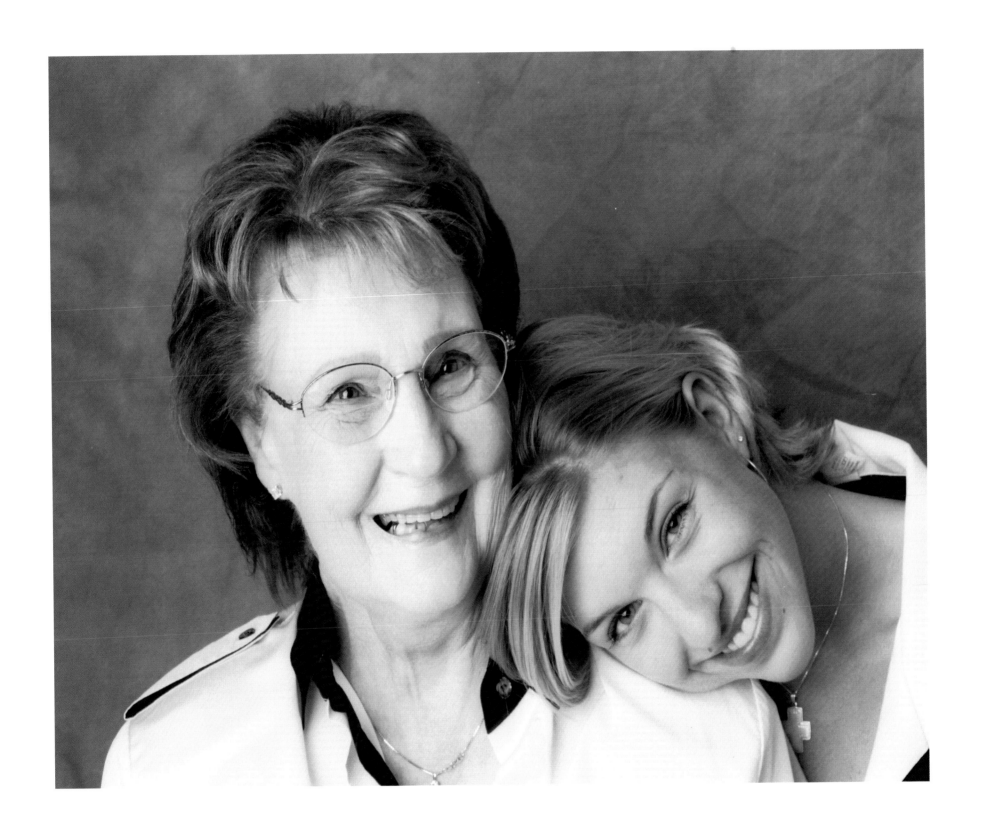

Deborah

Goddess of... New love, Motherhood and A New outlook on life

When I was diagnosed with **right breast cancer,** I was only **36 years old.** At first the doctor did a lumpectomy, but the margins were not clear. Then, I had a second lumpectomy, and the margins were not clear AGAIN. I then started chemotherapy.

Trusting my instincts, I went for a second opinion and then a third opinion. I wanted to search for the truth. The doctor wanted to do a third lumpectomy.

I decided I would rather have a mastectomy with an immediate reconstruction... by a different doctor!!! He dug me out and filled me back up.

Today, the margins are clear!

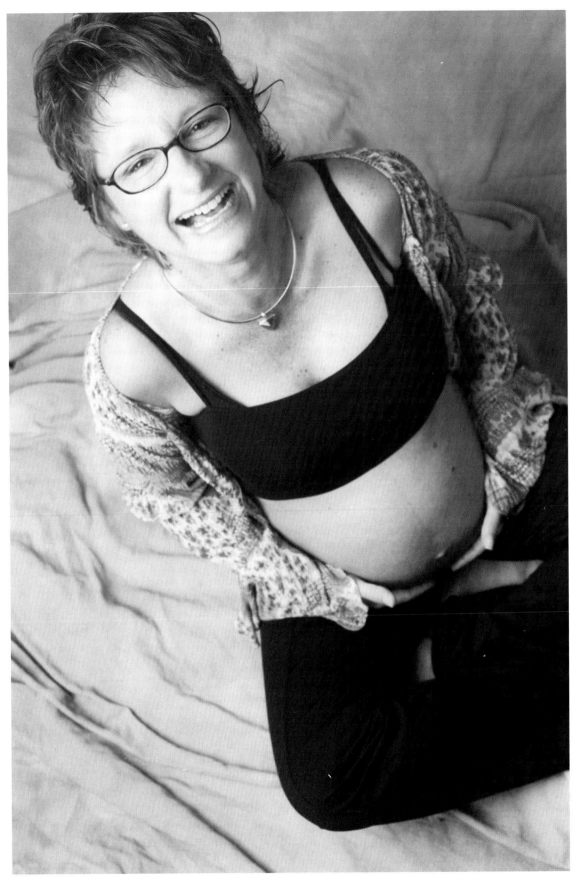

Deborah pregnant with Bay Ian

"Cancer has made me grounded."

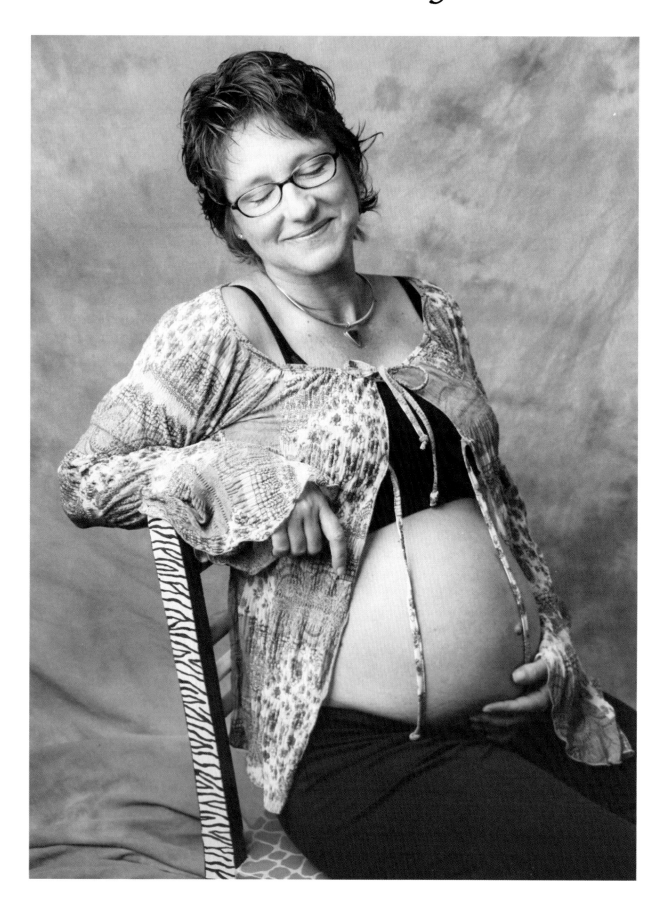

A love story
and a miracle...

I was invited to a party; I was bald and wore my usual scarf. I had an expensive wig ($400.00) but I never wore it. I felt relaxed at the party; it was a going-away celebration for a friend leaving for Germany.

Then HE walked in---we were caught in a moment. I turned back and saw Erich. Although I thought he was interested in my friend, I soon learned that he was checking me out. ME!!!! He watched me at the party and thought I had a great spirit. He saw through the scarf and my baldness.

Our first date was a exciting and memorable. He was a blast and he even wore my hat. We danced and socialized. That was it---**connection.** I tried to take it slowly...but **LOVE DOES NOT WAIT.**

I was told that the chemotherapy treatment made me sterile. It came as a pleasant surprise when two months later, we found out that I was pregnant with an angel-miracle-baby-boy. We have decided to name him Ian Daniel.

Previous to cancer, my life was in chaos. I was stressed out all the time and tired. My focus was drawn to unimportant things and I was consumed with bad energy.

Now I have my health, a wonderful man in my life and a baby on the way!

Judy
Goddess of... Giving and Honesty

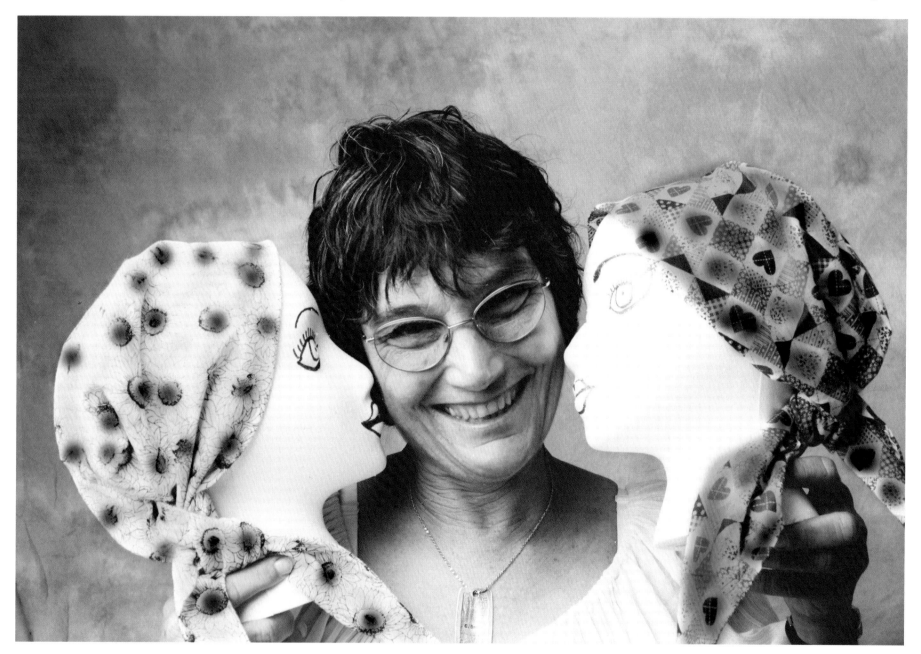

I have made over 2,500 scarves

(and donated all of them)

I love to share!

I was diagnosed with breast cancer almost ten years ago. I had chemotherapy and radiation.
Cancer DID change me. I am much more aware of how many people are affected by this disease.
Cancer reaffirmed my inner-strength. I now know that I am a survivor.

I used to be a high school physical education teacher. When I got cancer, I was honest with my students.
The greatest gift you can give--- is honesty. My students accepted what I was going through and understood
that I would be losing my hair. I did not wear a wig and I made my own scarves. I liked goofy hats and I
had one that said, "Bad Hair Day."

I like to share. I enjoy reaching out to others that need me.

I hand sew and donate cotton scarves for those that have lost their hair from chemotherapy.
I like knowing that I can make a difference. Making a scarf lets a women who shy about her baldness,
able to wear a pretty scarf and have some public ccomfort.

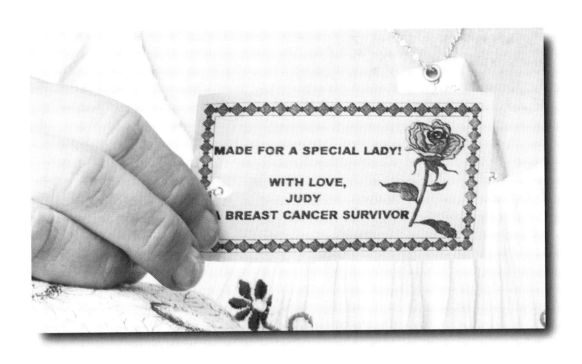

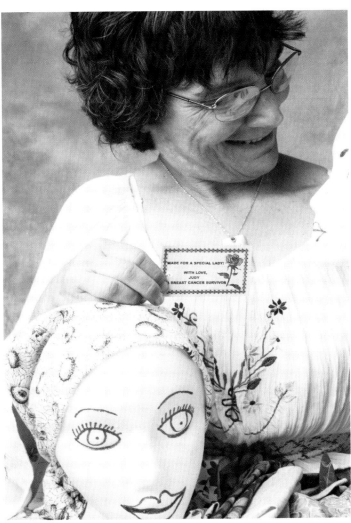

Goddess of... Independence and Perception

In October of 2000, I ran in a marathon in Dublin, Ireland. I was in terrific shape, having trained diligently all year for the event. Finishing the marathon was one of the highest moments of my life.

When I returned home, I was having difficulty breathing and had a nagging cough. I thought I had a respiratory infection from the cold, damp weather in Ireland. Four months later, the breathing difficulty had gotten worse and I was wheezing and it was a struggle just to walk up a flight of stairs. My doctor called it pleural effusion. He had a very seirous look on his face and said, "We'll need to run some more tests."

I went numb when he said the word "cancer."

Numerous tests and scans later, it was determined that I had **ovarian cancer**. It was found on an ultrasound. My surgery was scheduled for two weeks later. My doctor said, "Are you aware what's happening to you?" I was STILL numb.

Thirty days later I had surgery: radical hysterectomy (uterus and ovaries), appendectomy, 1 foot of my colon removed and parts of my liver. I had stage IV ovarian cancer. The cancer had spread to many organs, including my lymph nodes. My surgery was extensive, and recovery was hard. My days in the hospital were a blur of pain and sadness, dulled by painkillers. I barely had time to catch my breath when they administered the first chemotherapy treatment.

Chemotherapy was devastating. I felt so sick some days that I never moved out of bed. My hair fell out so fast and I was afraid to go out for fear of getting sick. I felt people staring at me and I hated their curious glances. I hated the way the rest of the world went on happily; I was trapped in my own world of pain, fear, and misery.

The bright spot of all was my support group: my parents, children and friends. My mother had been through cancer before, so she knew what I was going through and was so caring. I wouldn't have made it without her. My children were the shining lights in my dark world, just seeing their beautiful faces gave me a reason to try to get well.

After six rounds of chemotherapy and a brief four-month remission, the cancer came back. I was scheduled for another six rounds of chemotherapy. NOT FAIR!

Finally, chemotherapy was finished for the second time. My hair grew in and I started to feel a bit more normal. But... my life has changed forever. The thing I want so much is the thing that I will never have- my old life back. My friends treat me differently—almost as if I am a damaged good. I guess in some ways I am.

I know I need to learn to move forward and I will.

I feel I am entitled to be angry.
I am hurt when people run away from me.

Cancer has changed me forever....

But, I am stronger than it is!

Terry

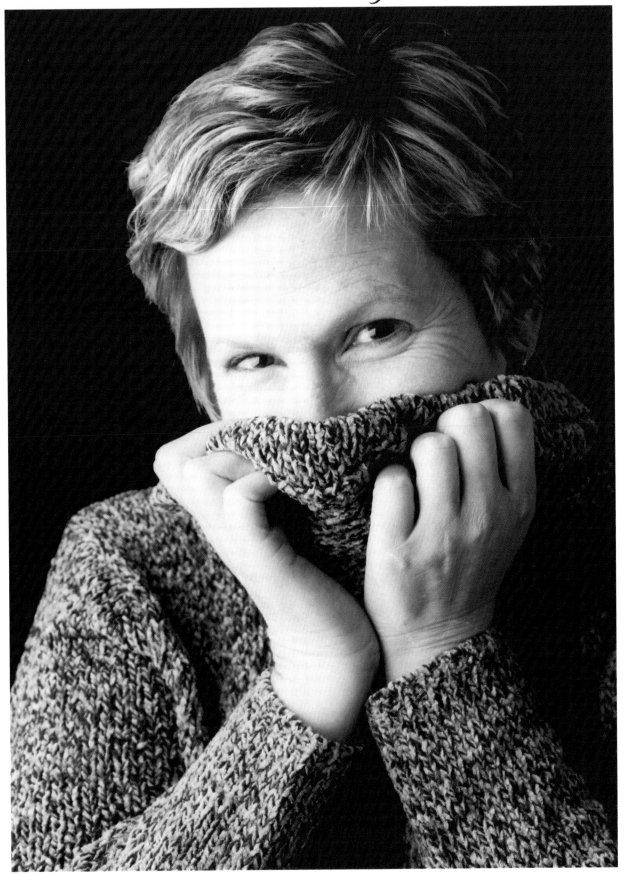

Independent vs. needy

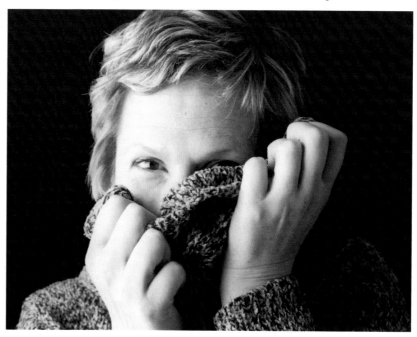

Expressive vs. running away

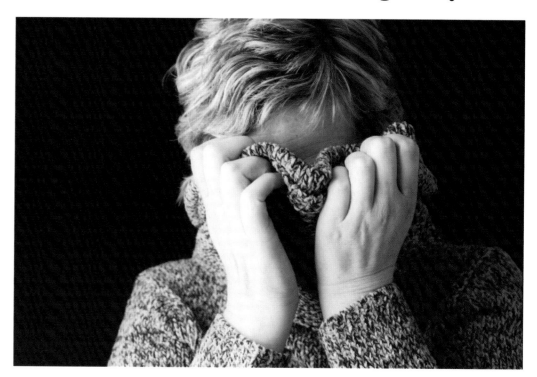

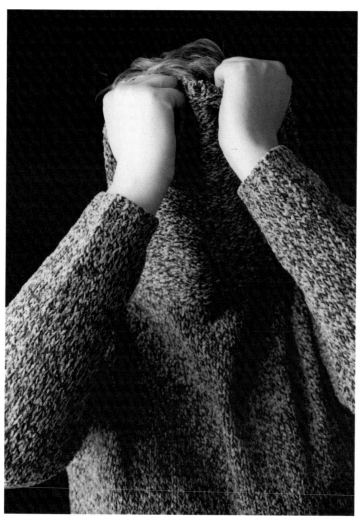

Wise vs. irrational

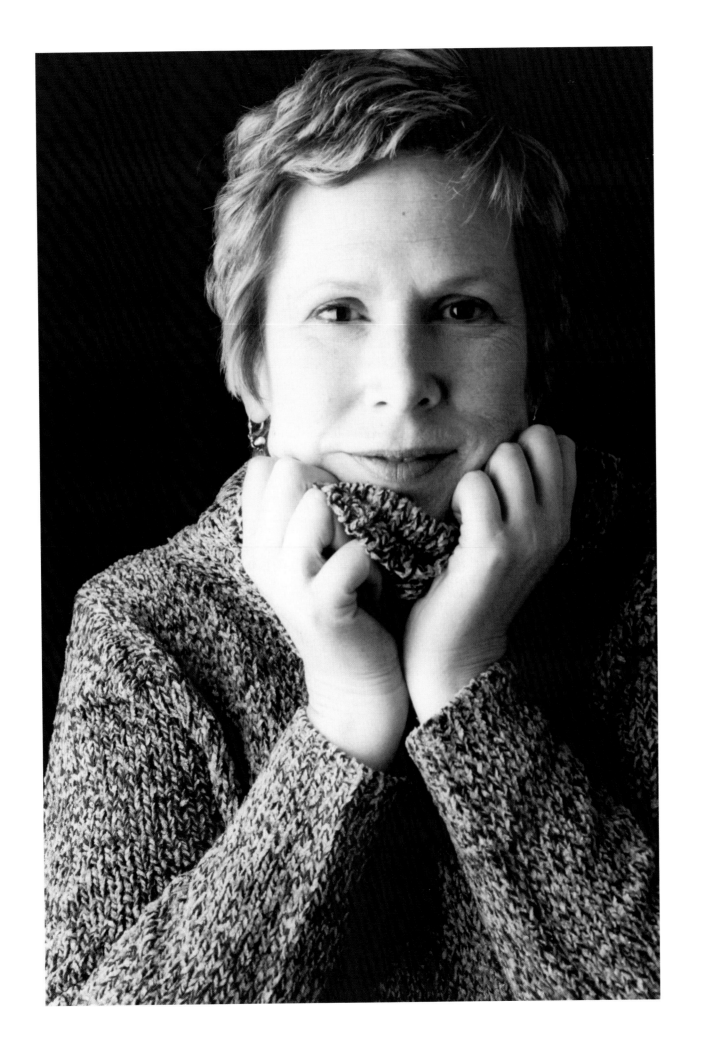

Joy

Goddess of... Marine Mammals and

The courage to tell her story to the world

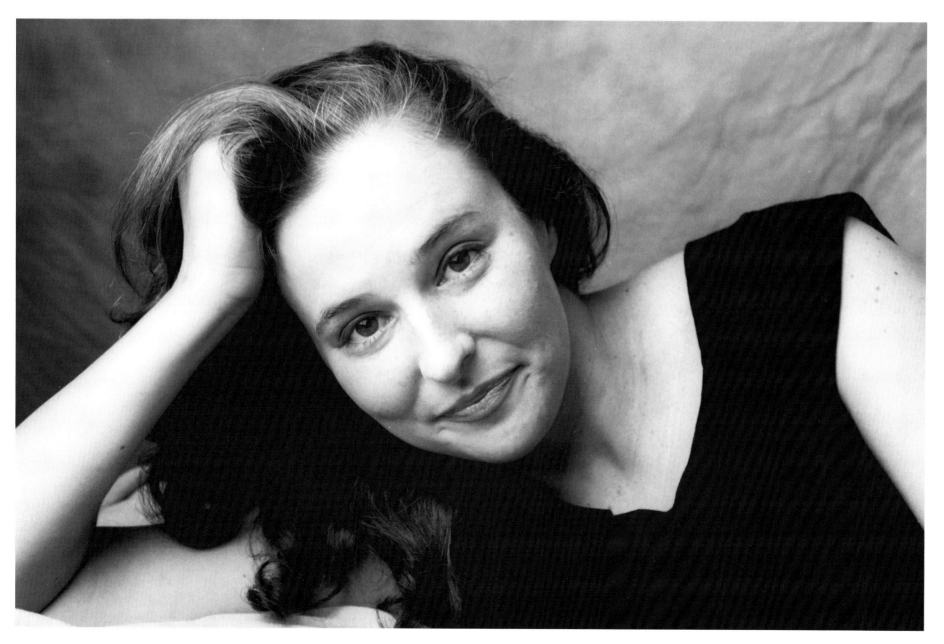

I was diagnosed with Non Hodgkin's Lymphoma (aggressive, Large B-cell), when I was 25 years old. On Thanksgiving, there was a large lump on the left side of my neck. I went to the urgent care center and the doctor kept pushing on the lump. "Does this hurt?" he asked. It did not hurt. I had just read an article about Leukemia and decided to ask the doctor if that's what he thought I had. The doctor did not respond. There is nothing worse than when someone does not answer you.

I named my tumor Henry. I used to sing songs about him. I put the word TUMOR in place of other words in famous songs. Like the song, "Me and My *Shadow*" was now "Me and My *Tumor*." Or, "I'm gonna wash that *tumor* right out of my hair." I always joked around. Some people did not get my sense of humor. Some people can't deal with you when are funny about something they consider a serious situation.

At first I was diagnosed with Hodgkin's Lymphoma. I started treatment in my small town. I was told, "This is the good cancer."

I got a second opinion from Stanford and the pathology came back as Non-Hodgkin's Lymphoma. The aggressive variety-- otherwise know as "the-bad-one-to-have."

My aunt connected me to Dr. Siegel; an oncology specialist at Children's Hospital of Los Angeles. He wanted to treat me aggressively, as he would treat a pediatric patient; my youth could handle the intensity. So, I was admitted to Children's Hospital. I had chemotherapy for six months. I would have five days of treatments and a few weeks break in-between rounds. During that time, my white blood cell count dropped and I would received Neupogen. Then when my labs went back up, it was time for chemotherapy again.

Being in a children's hospital had many advantages. I could have friends spend the night and always had tons of visitors. Everyone that worked there was so nice and made everything so much less scary.

When I first got sick, I decided to record the whole experience with my video camera. I was a film student at the time, so what could be better? The documentation began right away. I had never seen anyone else my age with cancer or witnessed their story. I wanted to show what it was like from a patient's point of view.

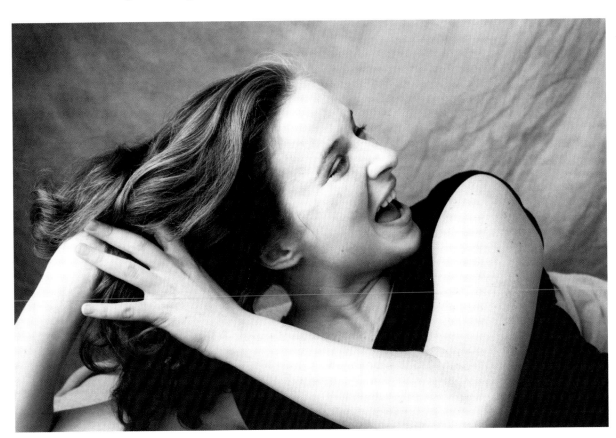

There are two points-of-view in my video. One aspect is the humorous times and the other is just reality, like when I had treatments and got my head shaved and so on. When I was alone, I would turn the video monitor around and look at myself in the screen. I would turn the camera on and talk to it. It became my journal, my friend and my confidant. I was always trying to be up and happy for my friends and family, I did not want to bring people down. To the camera, I could be sad, angry and brutally honest.

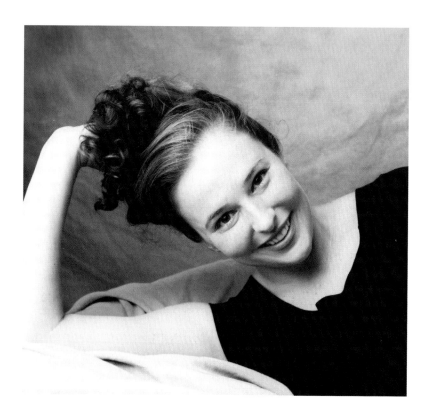

My friends did a lot of the filming for me. Pretty much anyone that would hold the camera got to film. Now I am editing the entire video. I have a cool program on the computer that I taught myself to use. I want to take the video to medical schools and show the doctors the patient's perspective of being treated for cancer. I want to demonstrate the humor and the pain.

The first doctor that treated me did not listen to me. She did not react to my illness or validate my feelings. My idea of a perfect doctor is one that can empathize and be sensitive. A lot of this has been lost. "I am fine," can really mean, "I am scared" or "I am going to throw-up" or "I feel like crap."

Other people's moods affect me; they are contagious. If someone is sad, they can bring me down too.

It has been two and a half years of being cancer free. This is a scary time, because this is the opportunity that it can return. At first I was worried and obsessed about being worried. Right now, since I feel so good, I am not scared.

Since I have had cancer, I have realized just how many people love me. My friends would call me on the phone and say, "I'll take some of your pain for you." We would concentrate really hard and the next day they would swear that their neck hurt. It was so amazing.

I am proud of being a cancer survivor. I can see myself standing on top of a mountain and screaming, "I survived!" I want to do this so that the subject is out in the open. I am a cancer survivor and I am proud and I want to talk about this. It's who I am now. I want people to be comfortable and feel open with me.

Now I am a little lost. I have a Bachelor's degree and a Master's degree in Social Sciences. I volunteered as a Hawaiian monk seal trainer and interned at Kewalo Basin Marine Mammal Lab. I was a professional dolphin trainer and then I became a professional cancer patient. I don't know what I am right now.

I feel like I was picked up out of the world and asked to fight for my life and then dropped back in to it. I am trying to re-enter.

My documentary is called: *Just One Year*-- It's an acronym for J.O.Y., my name.
My aunt thought of that.

It's time to get my story out there. I am ready, perhaps I just need a little push, but...   I have the power!

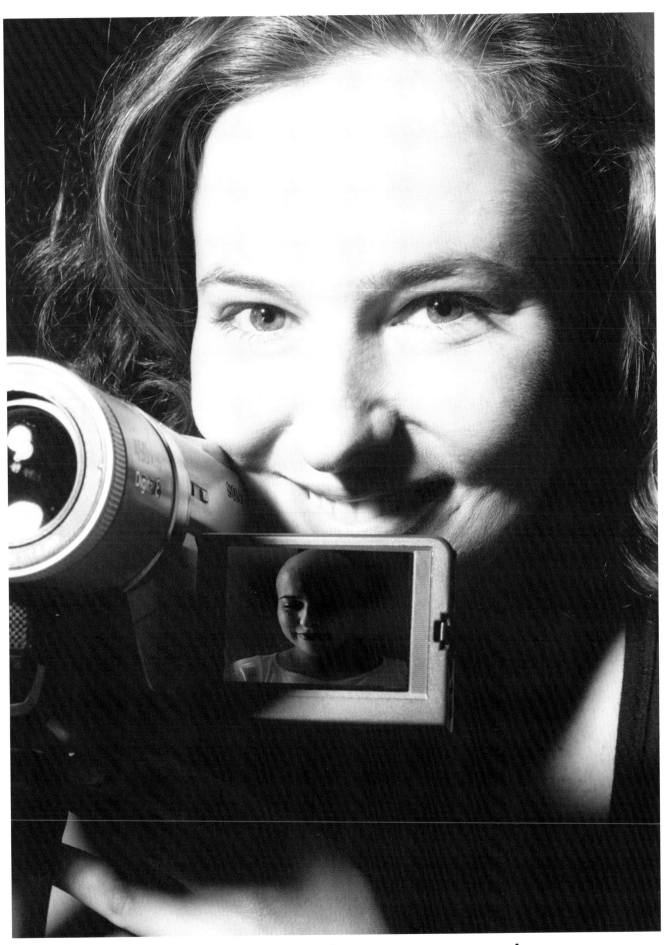

I video taped my entire cancer experience.

Thuy

Goddess of …Fighting and Recognizing her mission in life!

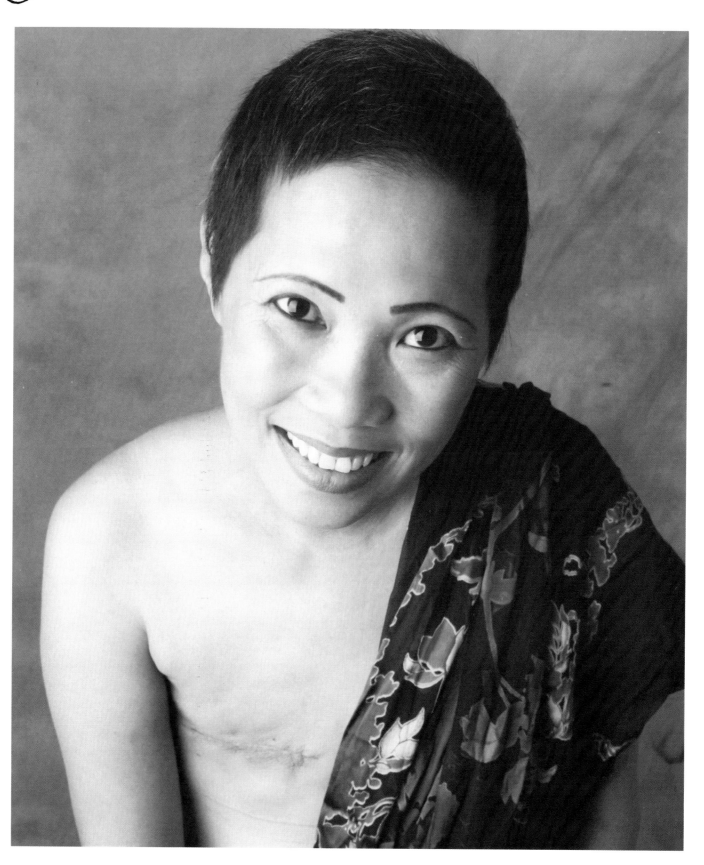

I am 42 years old. I am Vietnamese, but I live in the USA. I am married with three sons, they are: 10, 5 and 3 years old

I went to the doctor because I was having painful periods. I would just curl up and cry. By the time I went the the doctor, my abdomen was so swollen. I looked six months pregnant. The doctor came into the room and he shut the door. He told me to have a seat. He told me that I had cancer. I was shocked. I was stunned. Then, I just had no reaction at all. I was frozen. The doctor said, "It's okay to cry."

Then, I was diagnosed with **ovarian cancer, stage III**. I had a total hysterectomy done right away.

One month laster I had a bowel obstruction. The adhesions from the surgery caused this problem. I had to have another surgery to remove six feet of my intestines and six inches of my colon.

A few months laster, I found a lump in my right breast. I had a lumpectomy. There were 13 lymph nodes removed and seven were positive for cancer.

Then, I had a right radical mastectomy with radiation.

I have had 10 rounds of chemotherapy for the ovarian cancer.
I have had 5 surgeries on my breast.
I have had 7 weeks of radiation.

I am now on hormone replacement.

My body has been through a lot.

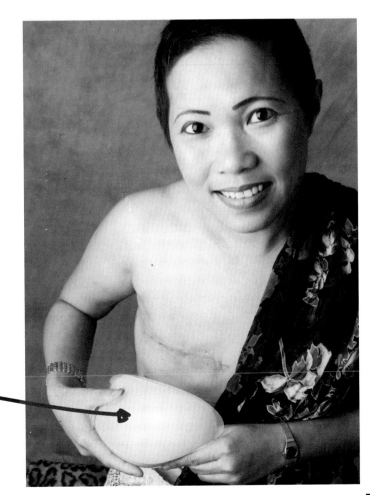

A breast prosthetic for my bra

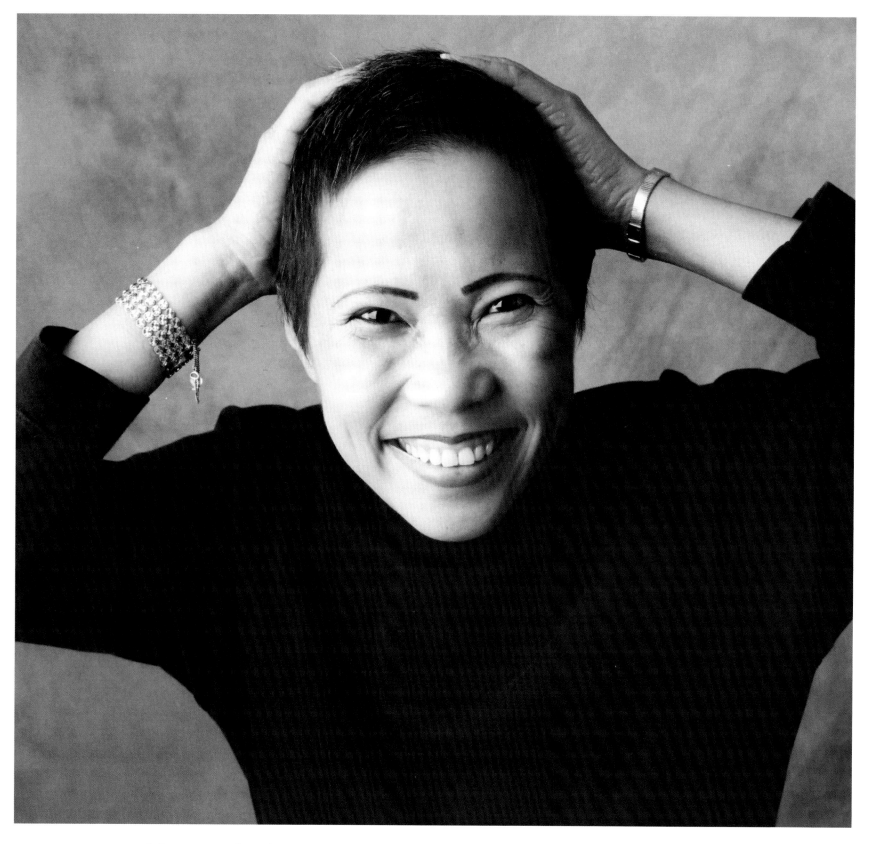

" I enjoyed being bald. When I wore a wig...my kids laughed at me."

I have the family stresses of the Eastern Medical Philiosophy, but I am in the USA and completely absorbed in Western medicine. My mom wanted me to take Chinese herbs, but I stopped.

When I got sick, I wanted to make a will with my husband. He refused. The Vietnemese culture says, *"Don't talk about it- then it won't happen."*

I love to eat. I am a fighter. I know my mission in life is to raise my sons. They need their mom. I need them. I am not done living.

I worship Buddha and have a shrine at home. I sit there for comfort and talk silently to God or some higher power. I light candles and bring flowers to the alter.

I would say I am uptight and easily stressed.

Most of my support comes from the people I work with. There is a friend at work who participated in the "Avon Three Day Breast Cancer Walk" in my honor. I was so touched by this.

Recently I was informed that I carry the breast cancer gene. This means that the cancer will most likely return to my other breast. I have to make a tough decision now: do I remove my other breast before the cancer strikes?

I would like reconstruction because I would feel like a whole person. When I dress up in a gown for a formal party, I do not have the cleavage to fill out the top part of the dress. I start to feel self conscious. Then again, how often do I wear fancy clothes? Is cleavage really that important? I am not in my 20's looking for a date. I am a mom and a wife, but I still want to feel sexy. I cannot make a decision right now.

Holly

Goddess of ... Importance and Motherhood

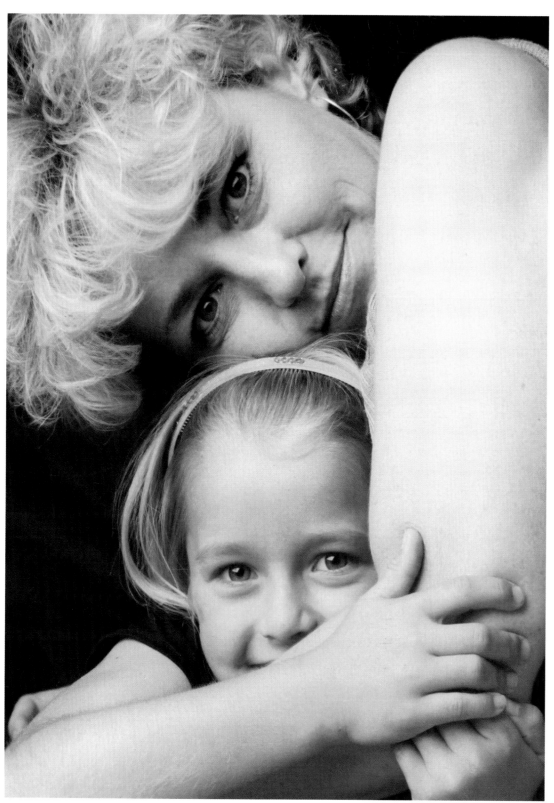

Holly and Kate

My daugher Kate is wonderful. I grew up with a stepmom, my real mom was a mess and left our family (seven kids) when I was five years old. When I was diagnosed with cancer, Kate was five years old.

Surviving became the most important thing to me. I did not want my daughter to grow up without a mom. I could not die, I could not leave her!

On January 10, I was diagnosed with right breast cancer. I had surgery and they removed 18 lymph nodes and I had a full mastectomy. I had chemotherapy and radiation.

On March 3, I started reconstructive surgery. I am still not happy with my new breast. The implant feels weird. I will have it redone someday.

I have been married 11 years to Troy. He held my hand during every chemotherapy treatment. Losing my hair was more traumatic than losing my breast. I used to have straight blonde hair. Now it's out of control and curly.

We never know how much time we have!

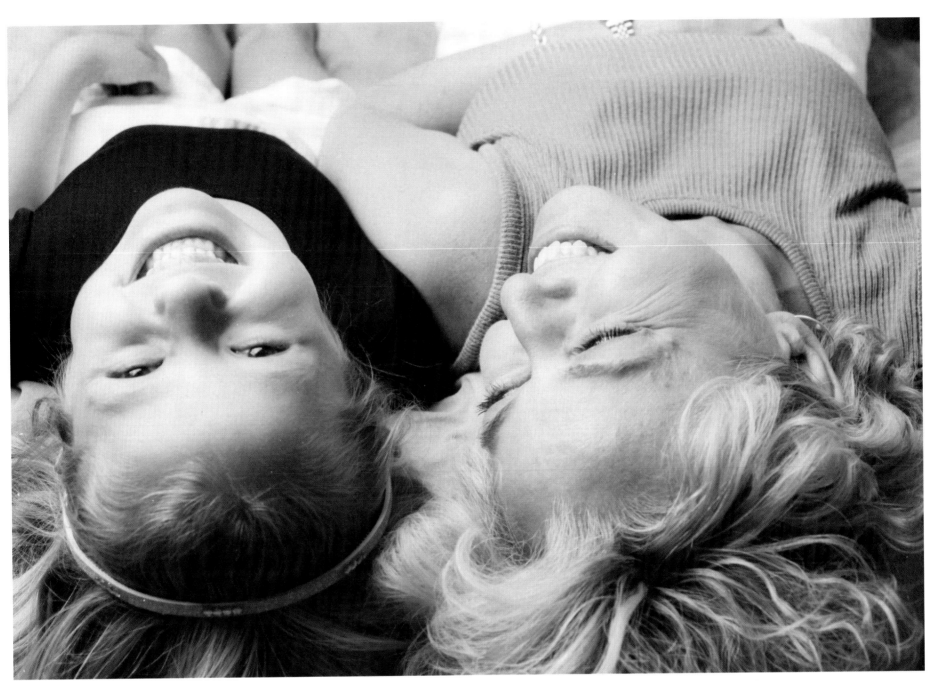

Cancer is a wakeup call, not a death sentence!

Rebecca *Goddess of... Art and Forgiving*

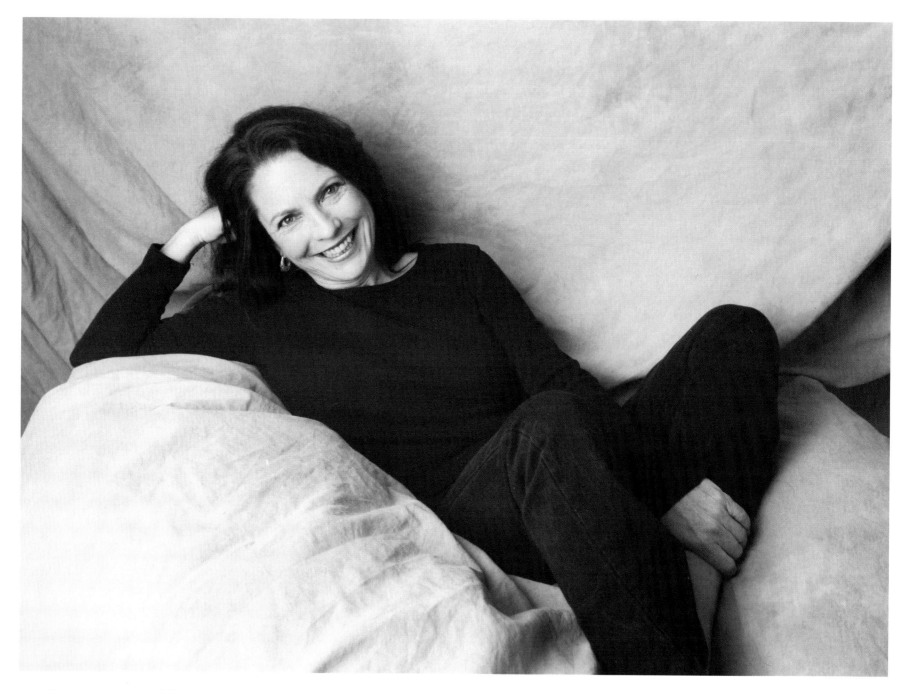

I am a 51-year-old artist! (Painting & Drawing) At 30 I had cervical cancer and had a total hysterectomy.
On December 31st, I was diagnosed with right breast cancer (Sentinel Node)
I was fatalistic at the beginning, but I was able to see the light. I opted for what is considered "conservative"
therapy: lumpectomy, radiation and Tomaxifan for five years.
I was living in Hawaii; I had not allowed time to pursue a profession as a painter. I said to myself, "What the hell?!"
I moved back to California and started my career as an artist. While recovering, I received a grant to attend
the Academy Art College in San Francisco. I have won several awards for my paintings.
One year after my encounter with breast cancer, my younger sister was diagnosed with breast cancer.
I thought, "Of all people? This is not right! I already had cancer, leave her alone!"
Thankfully--we are both in remission.

Today: I don't carry anger and it is easier for me to forgive others.

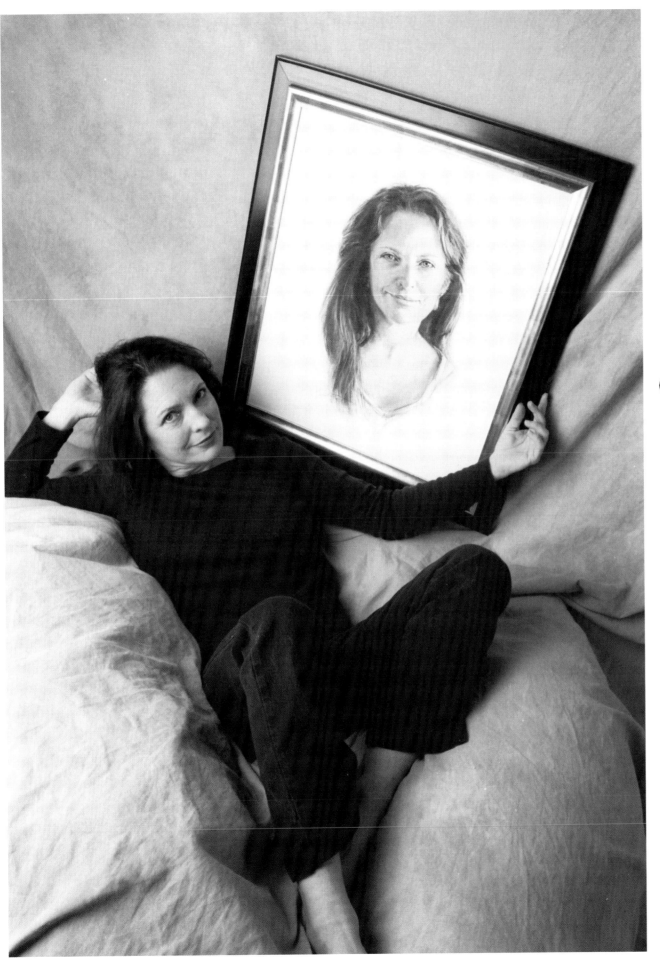

Self Portrait

HOLLY & REBECCA

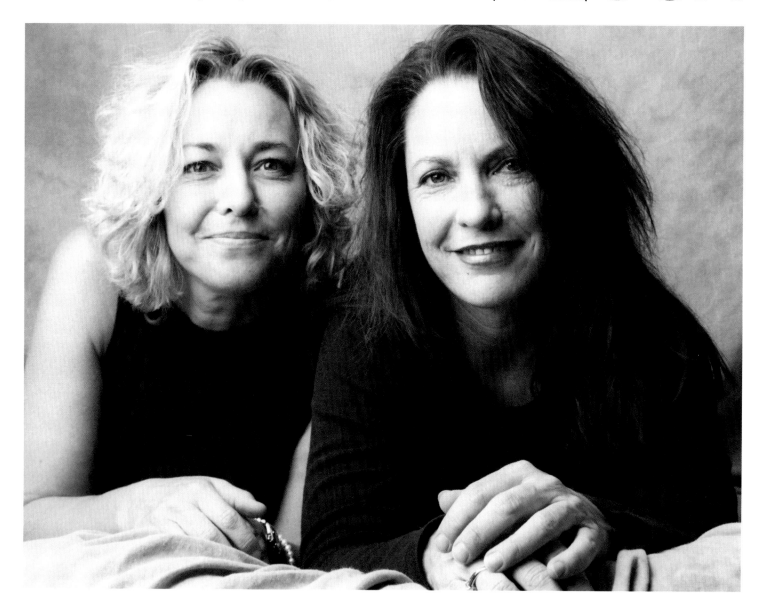

THE SISTERS OF SURVIVAL!

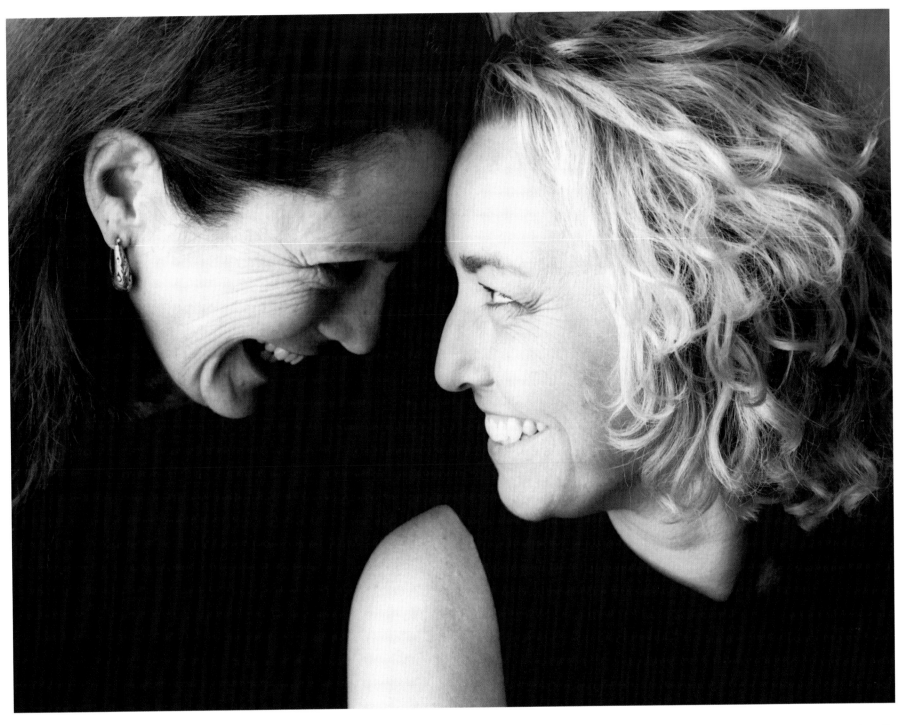

Rebecca and Holly

"Some are born great, some achieve greatness, and some have greatness thrust upon 'em." --William Shakespeare

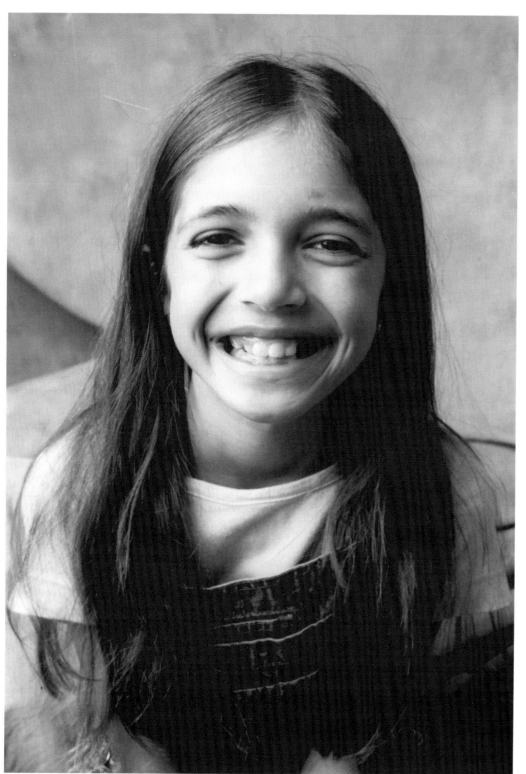

Lindsay
Goddess of generosity

At ten years old, Lindsay cut 10 inches of her hair and donated it to the organization called "Locks Of Love."

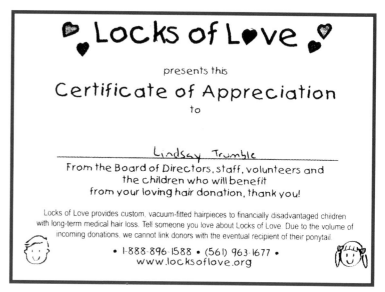

Locks of Love

presents this

Certificate of Appreciation

to

Lindsay Trumble

From the Board of Directors, staff, volunteers and the children who will benefit from your loving hair donation, thank you!

Locks of Love provides custom, vacuum-fitted hairpieces to financially disadvantaged children with long-term medical hair loss. Tell someone you love about Locks of Love. Due to the volume of incoming donations, we cannot link donors with the eventual recipient of their ponytail.

• 1-888-896-1588 • (561) 963-1677 •
www.locksoflove.org

"Locks of Love" is a non-profit organization that provides hairpieces to financially disadvantaged children under the age of 18 suffering from long-term medical hair loss. They meet a unique need for children by using donated hair to create the highest quality hair prostetics. The wigs they provide help to restore self-esteem and confidence, enabling children to face the world and their peers. They accept a minimum of 10 inches of hair. The majority of hair donated comes from other children.

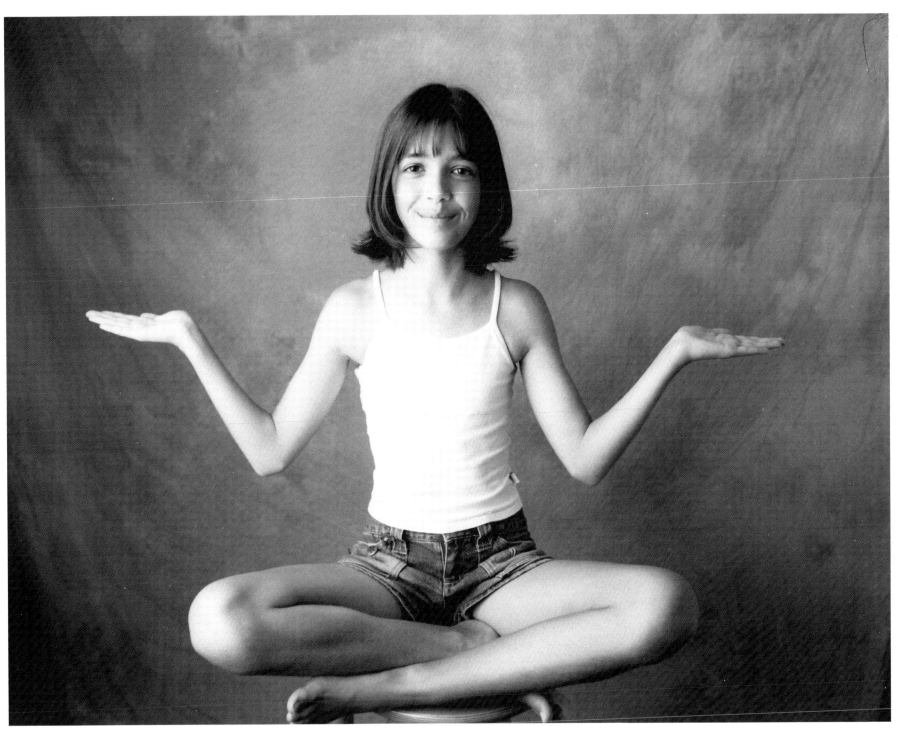

Lindsay shows off her new hairdo after cutting ten inches of her hair and donating it to "The Locks of Love" organization.

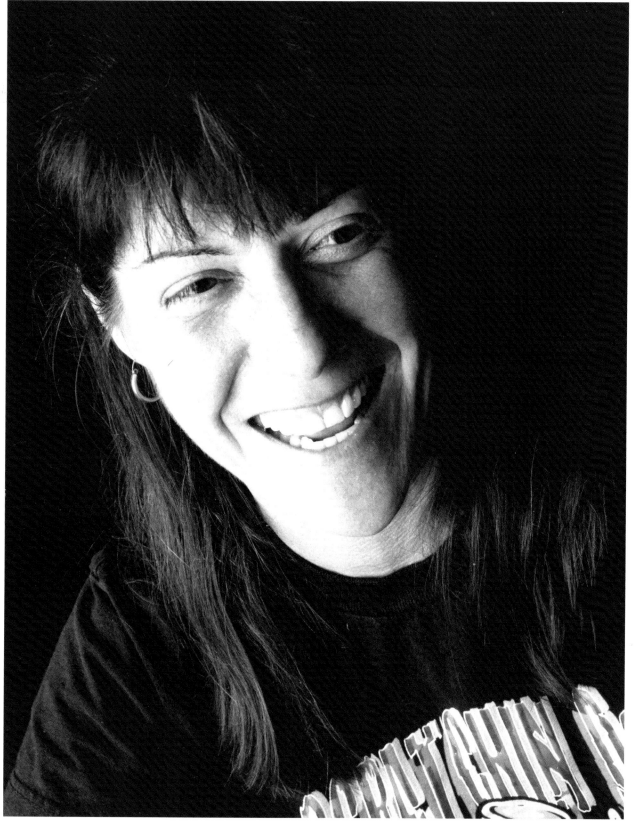

LINDA

Goddess of... Pride!

I was brought up never to feel sorry for myself.

I have Chronic Lymphocytic Leukemia (CLL). This means that I have cancer of the white blood cells and bone marrow. My body makes too many immature white blood cells, and these cells do not perform their normal fuctions, plus they take up the room of the functioning cells. My symptoms include: enlarged lymph nodes, elow platelets, fatigue and

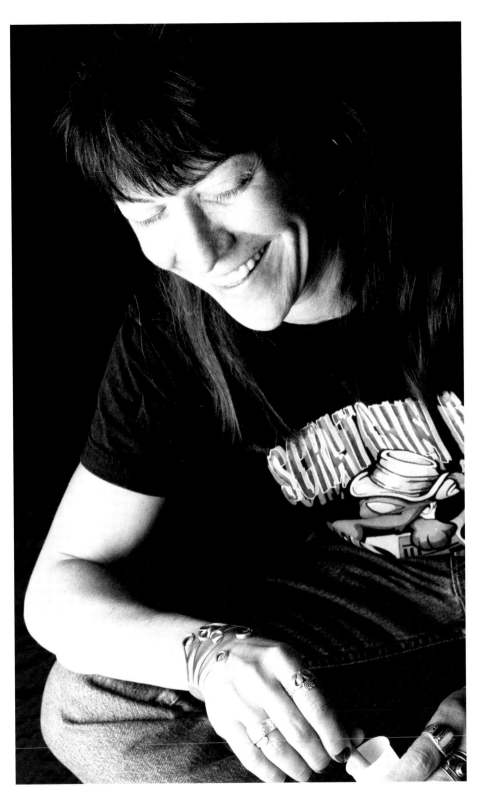

severe bone pain. I feel physically exhausted but mentally charged, like a little kid that has been swimming all day long, in the sun, I try to sleep at night, but my mind will not turn off. There are days when I have no energy at all.

I went gone to the doctor because I had been feeling so sick. I was tired and my entire body hurt. I felt like I had the flu. When the doctor told me I had cancer, in some way, I was relieved that there was a name that would explain the way I had been feeling.

I do not have medical insurance. I have read that the survival rate for those that don't have insurance goes down

I qualify for M.I.A, which stands for *Medical Indigent Adult*. With a name like that, it sounds like you are *a loser*. The program is for people who are uninsured and who are not eligible for other health care coverage. MIA helps me get medical care by paying for all or part of the cost. This is a county funded program. They help with my medical bills, and pay for the routine blood work I need and most of the medications that I have to take. I am so thankful for any help that I can get.

I have received chemotherapy, steroids and Rituxan. Now I have *residual disease*-- a fancy term for something that confuses me. Since there is no cure, I have to live with the day-to-day side affects of the illness. Each day I feel differently, so it's hard to hold a typical Monday through Friday job. I can get up and feel great one morning or not get out of bed at all the next day. Because I am 39 years old, people expect me to be more energetic. I enjoyed working when I could.

The worst part of all of this... how low do you have to go in order to get some help? I do not have the usual privilages such as, a bank account, credit card or a car. If I did not have good friends, I would be homeless. I am so lucky to have my friends. Even though it's difficult to accept, it is nice to be loved and taken care of.

I am an artist. I love to paint.
There is a woman that is interested in my
work. She wants me to do a show. The
thought of displaying my work gives me
something positive to think about. I love to
express humor in my paintings.   Painting
gives my busy brain a break. I can
escape into another place, I just need a
canvas, my brushes and paint.

I have a tattoo that says; "Contentless Fear."
I had it done when I was younger. I sold
one of my paintings to pay for the tattoo.
At the time, I thought I was living a
contentless fear life. Now that I have
something to really be afraid of, I find
many more things to be content with.

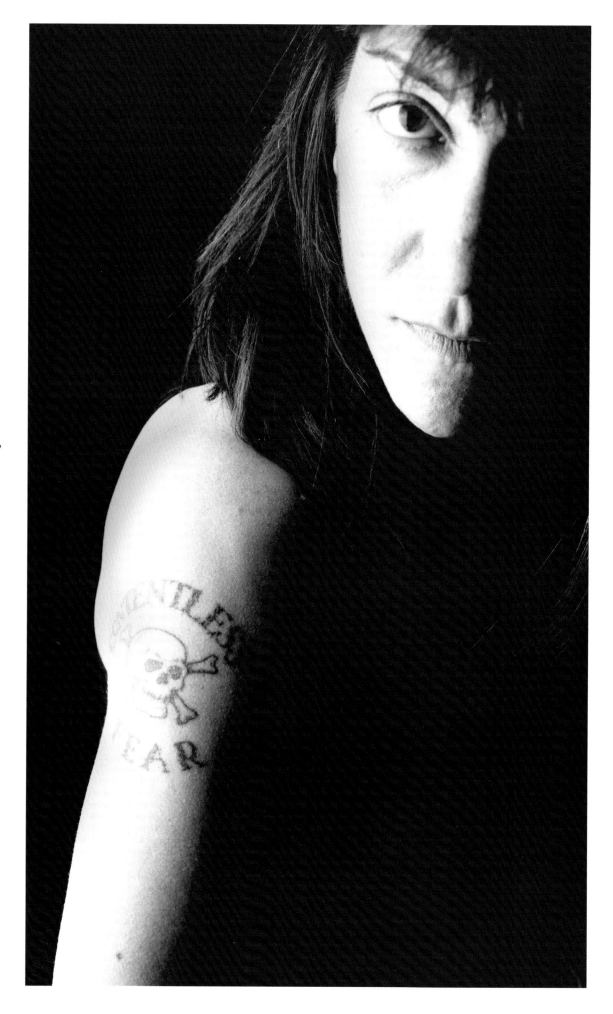

I am not the assertive type. My experience
with doctors is that they don't want to
answer your questions completely. If you
back them into a corner and insist on a straight
answer, then you might get one.   I asked one
of my doctors, "Why do I still have swollen
lymph nodes?"   His answer was, "Sometimes
things just don't work."

I am involved at the local cancer center. I can
get free relaxtion therapies and there is asupport
group for blood involved cancers. I look to my
support groups for the answers. Everyone
seems more open, right down to the core.

There is an imbalance between desperately wanting
the pain to subside and enduring the side affects
of the pain medications. A strong narcotic will take
the soreness away but side affect is drowsiness.
Added lethargy is not fun, especially since I am
already so tired to begin with.

I find passion in the smallest things. I love
my house plants and gave them all names,
Herzog and Dina. I put them outside during
the day, so they can absorb the sunlight.
At night, I bring them back inside.

I was not brought up to feel sorry for myself.
My family and friends give me the support I need.

I feel really lucky to have the love and
the encourgement from my friends.
I could not get through many days
without them. I do not have much, but
I am rich when it comes to friends.
My Friendships are immeasurable.

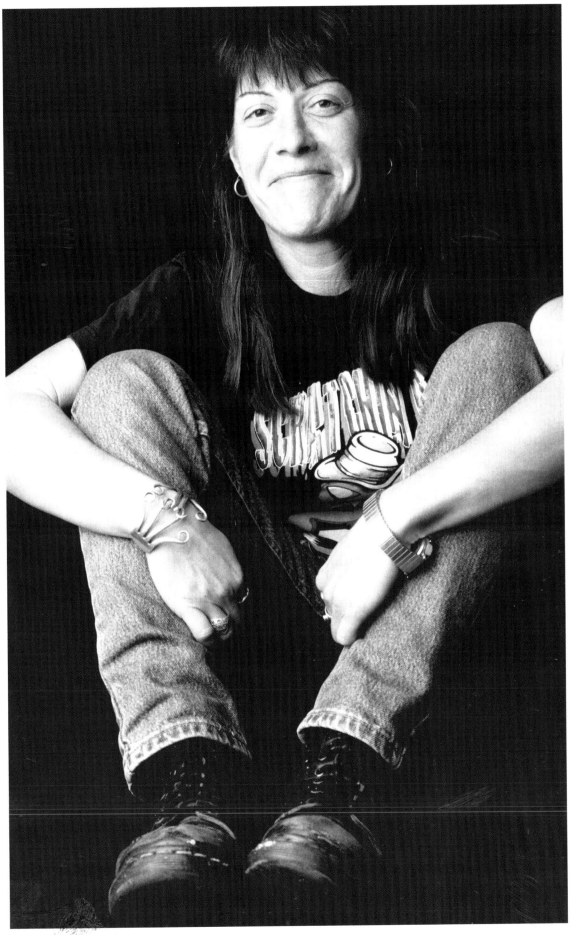

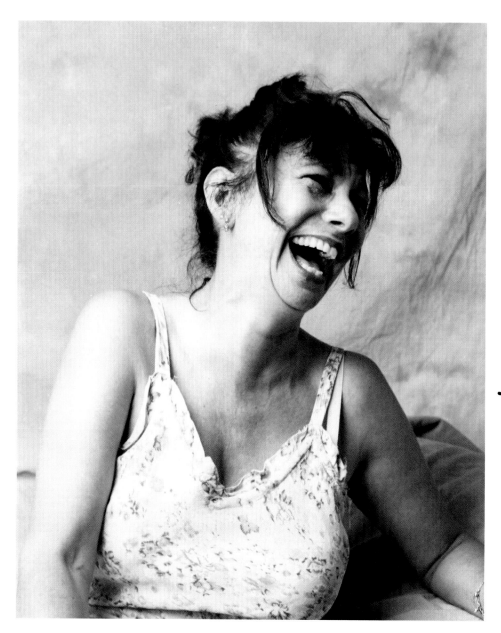

Diane

Goddess of...
Touch and Alternative Medicine

Prior to cancer, I taught first grade and was an aerobics instructor. I am a single mom of twin boys that are 21 years old. One attends Harvard, the other attends UCLA. Not bad, huh?

I was diagnosed with **breast cancer** three years ago. I thought, I can't bother being sick. (I do have a history of Lyme Disease and Chronic Fatigue Syndrome. I have a weak immune system).

I had a partial mastectomy. I have unevenly sized breasts. I like to refer to them as, Little Joe and Big Mama.

I have chosen holistic medicine for further treatments. I believe in accupuncture, medical Qi-Gong, herbs, oxygen therapy and Reiki. This is what works for me. I love to teach people about the alternative they can add to the more traditional Western practices (chemotherapy and radiation).

I am involved at the local cancer center where I am a certified Reiki Master.

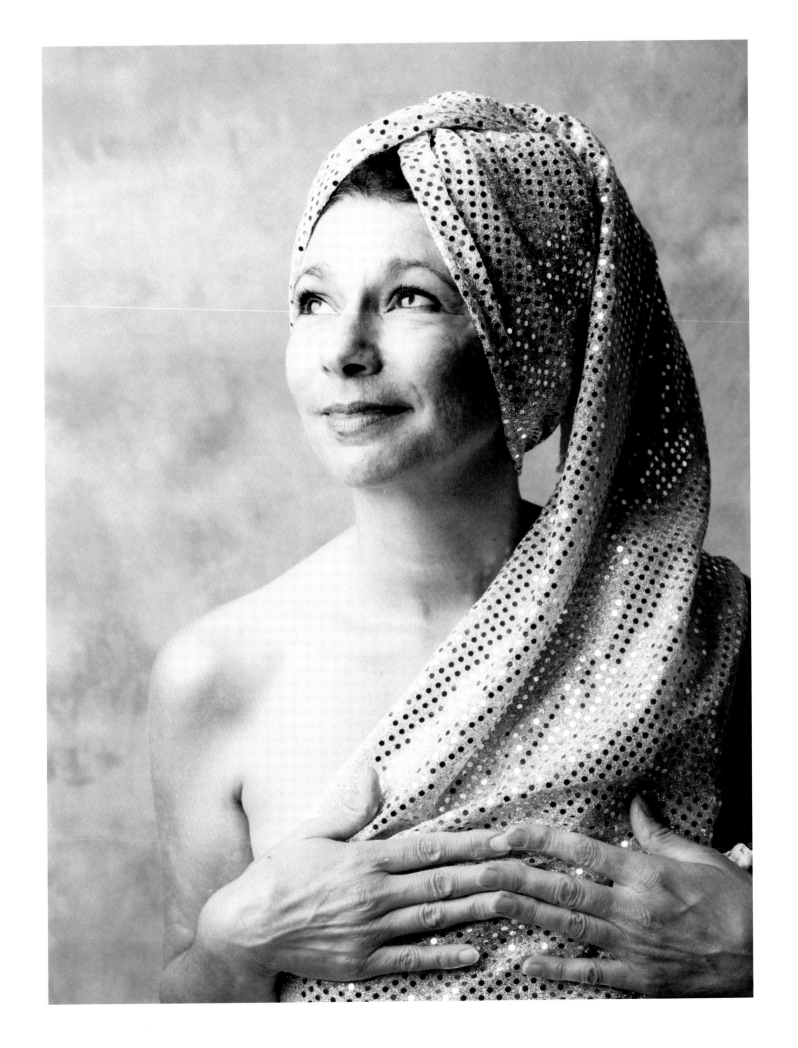

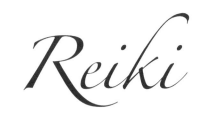

Reiki

Pronounced: Ray-Key

Definition: A method of natural healing based on the application of the *Universal Life of Energy*.

The word Reiki breaks down:
Rei: Universal life,
Ki: Energy.

Reiki is an ancient form of "laying on of hands" energy that is 2,500 years old. This is a Japanese tradition form of healing that attemps to equalize the energy imbalances in the body that can manifest as physical or emotional discomfort.

During a Reiki session, the patient does not undress. The patient lies on a comfortable spot (bed, massage table, etc.), the room is dimly light and there can be soft music playing. The environment should be relaxing. The Practioner places their hands on various positions of the body so the transmission of the *Reiki Energy* can begin to flow into the patient.

The core of the body (abdomen & chest) and the head are two primary sites of Reiki hand placement.

*On the opposite page, Diane demonstrates Reiki exersises that you can do on yourself.

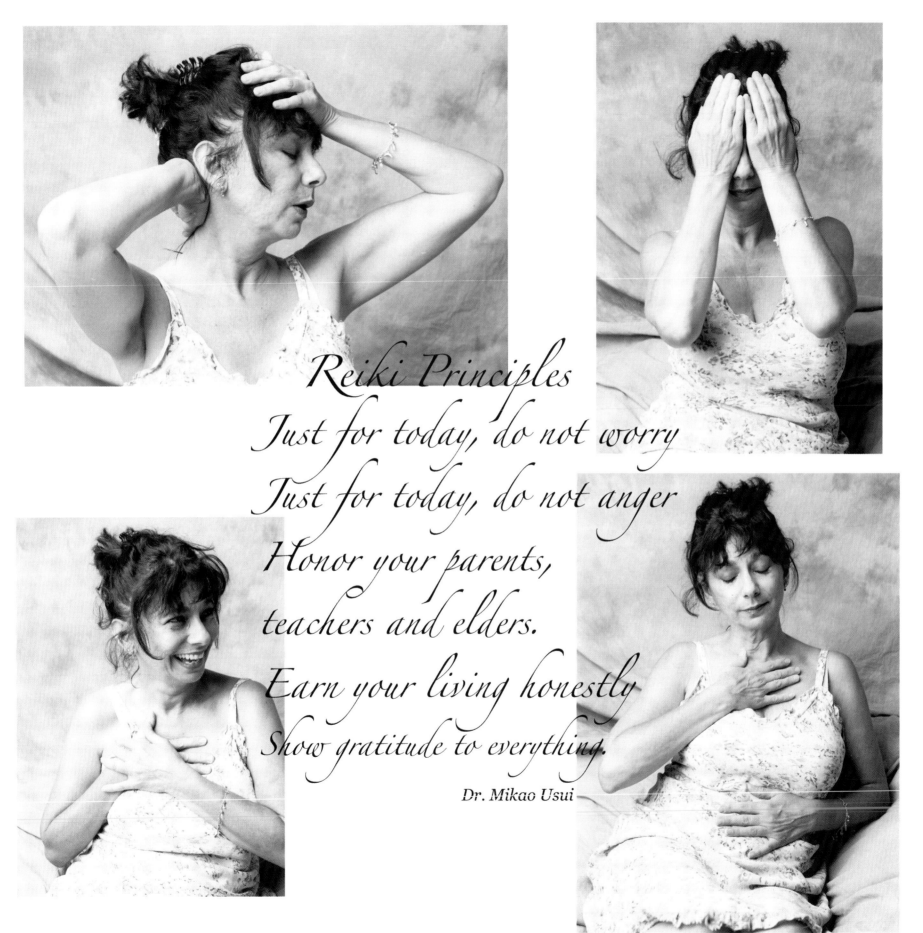

Reiki Principles

Just for today, do not worry

Just for today, do not anger

Honor your parents,

teachers and elders.

Earn your living honestly

Show gratitude to everything.

Dr. Mikao Usui

Eliane

Goddess of... Dancing and Radiating

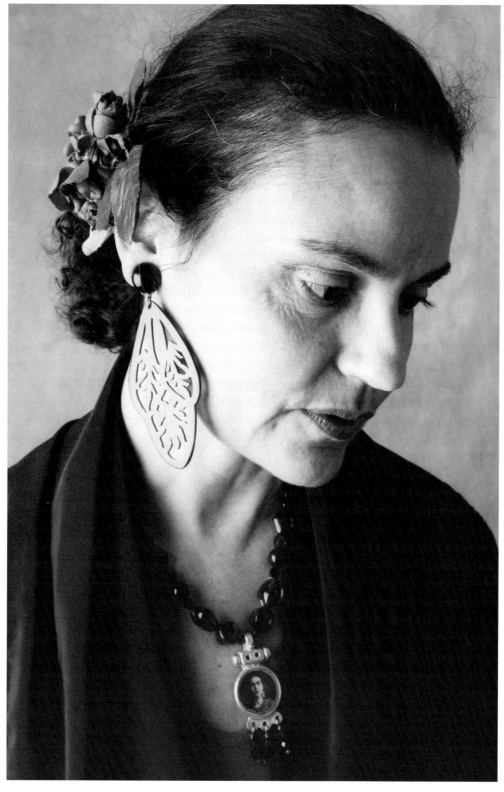

I am a breast cancer survivor. I love to dance- Flamenco style. When my soul is desperate, I just dance and the movements and the music bring me back.

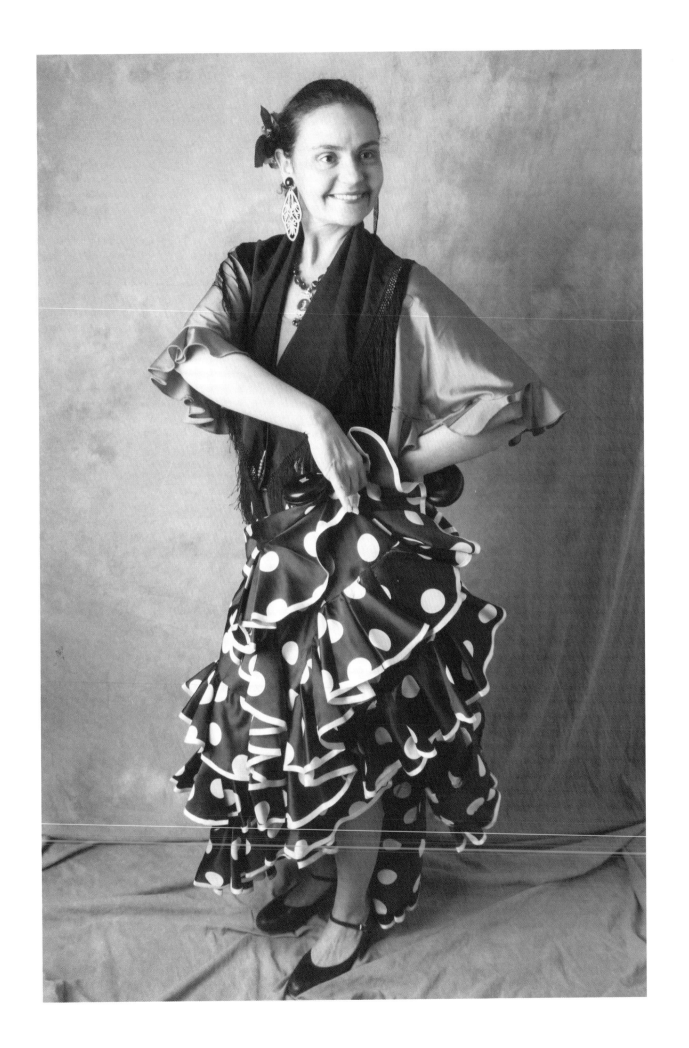

Jevine
Goddess of...Reading, Painting & Optimisim

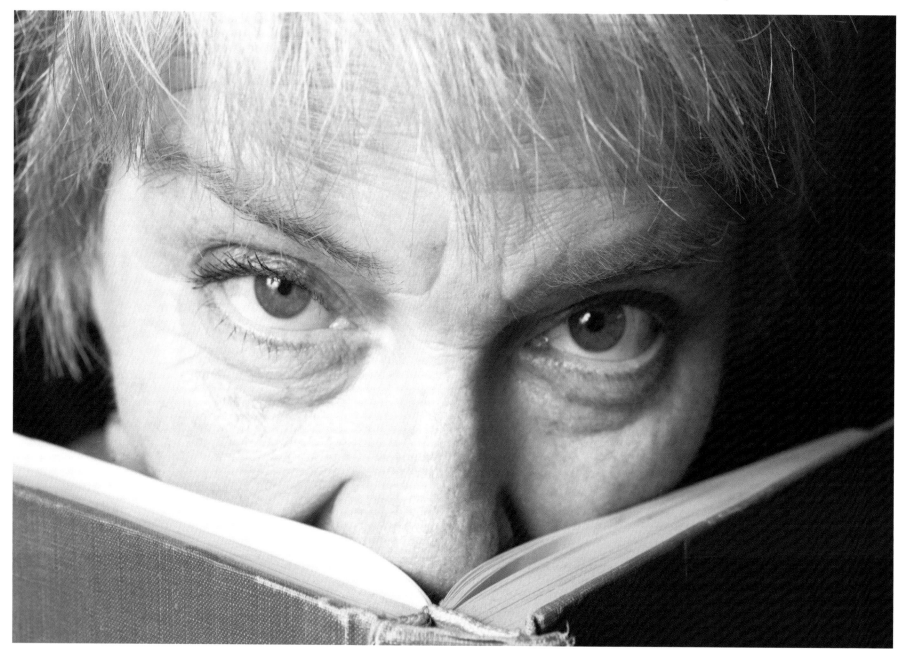

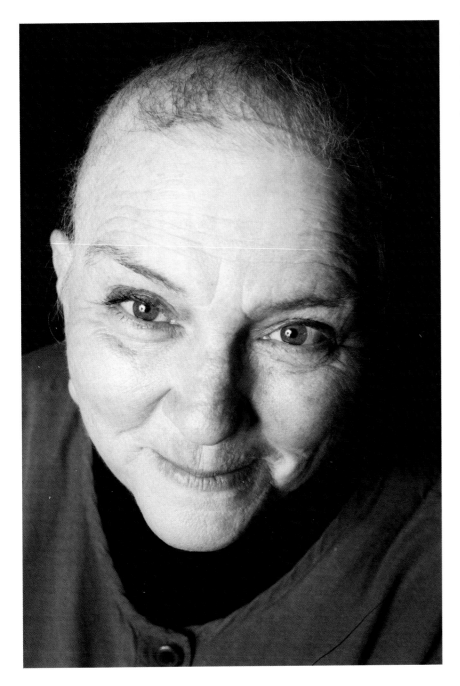

I am 67 years old and I have **lung cancer**. I had been complaing of shortness of breath and a sore throat for two years. Since these are common side affects that can be related to many illnesses, nobody appreared to be that worried. Then, I changed doctors and saw a Gastroenterologist; he took a different approach. The tests showed that I had a partially collapsed esophagus and the X-Ray showed where the cancer was.

I have small cell lymphoma, located on my lung. It was found at an early stage. Usually by the time cancer is found on the lungs, it's too late. **Early detection was good news!**

With cancer you lose two things: hair and friends. That's the bad news. Four and a half years ago, my husband Chris passed away suddenly. I was doing okay. I was on the path back to life and then along came cancer. My husband and I were married 40 years. I miss him! I know that if he had to watch me be sick, it would be hard on him. He was so sensitive and caring.

My chemotherapy treatments are three times a week for three weeks over a six month period. Then I will have radiation five days per week for seven weeks. When I am done with this, the doctors want to radiate my brain. They feel like if the cancer returns, it will go there. Supposedly chemotherapy does not cross the blood-brain-barrier and radiation is the only option as a preventative.

It is startling that the doctors do not know that much about my cancer and the treatment for it. My cancer is in such an early stage that it is an unfamiliar territory. I will have radiation on my chest, and this could damage my heart muscle or it could be fatal. I guess I am fatalistic at times. The radiation to my brain really scares me. I can lose my memory- how much memory is a mystery. The options are equally devastating: lose your memory or have cancer in your brain.

I have *chemo-brain; m*eaning, I am forgetful at times. This term is somewhat confusing, since the chemotherapy does not go to your brain. What are the long term effects? The doctors only want to talk about the cure and NOW. They do not talk about the rest of your life.

I have found an abundance of information about a lot of other cancers. I'll say to my doctor, "So, do I lose the taste in my mouth?" He'll say, "No, that happens with another kind of cancer." It's kind of a funny thing.

Right now, I am helping out at my daughter's used bookstore in Santa Barbara. I love to read. I love to get lost in books. I am lucky that I have some dear friends and family nearby. I have five children who are encouraging and sensitive.

You must do the things you want to do, at any time! I paint and sing jazz.
Lately, I cannot perform in crowded places. I am susceptible to germs in closed and crowded rooms. I am hungry for music.

I have been craving carbohydrates like crazy.
I will want to eat a big, fat hamburger and a side of onion rings. YUMMY.

Right now, I need to get in touch with how I really feel.
I have sorrow, frustration and hope.
I have gratitude for my friends and family.
I would like to find a support group.
I attended one after my husband died and it was invaluable.

There are things that I need to live for.
I have a granddaughter who is named after me- Emma Jevine. She's three months old and precious.

I want everyone to know that I am going to get well.

I know that lung cancer is
often associated with death...

I will survive this!

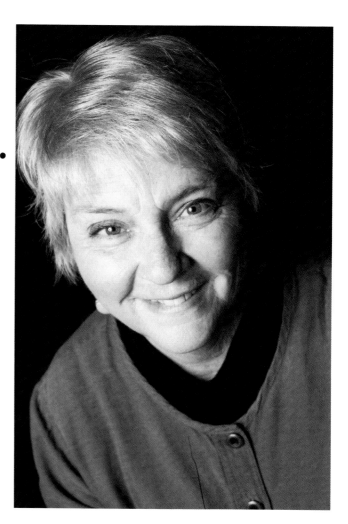

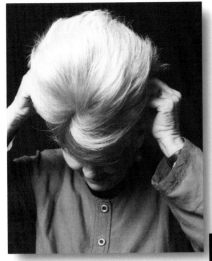

1

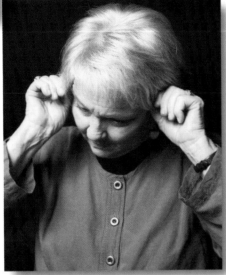

2

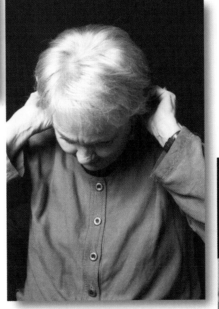

3

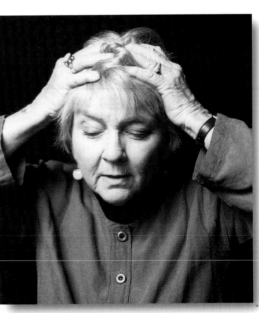

4

Helen

Goddess of... Reality and Purpose

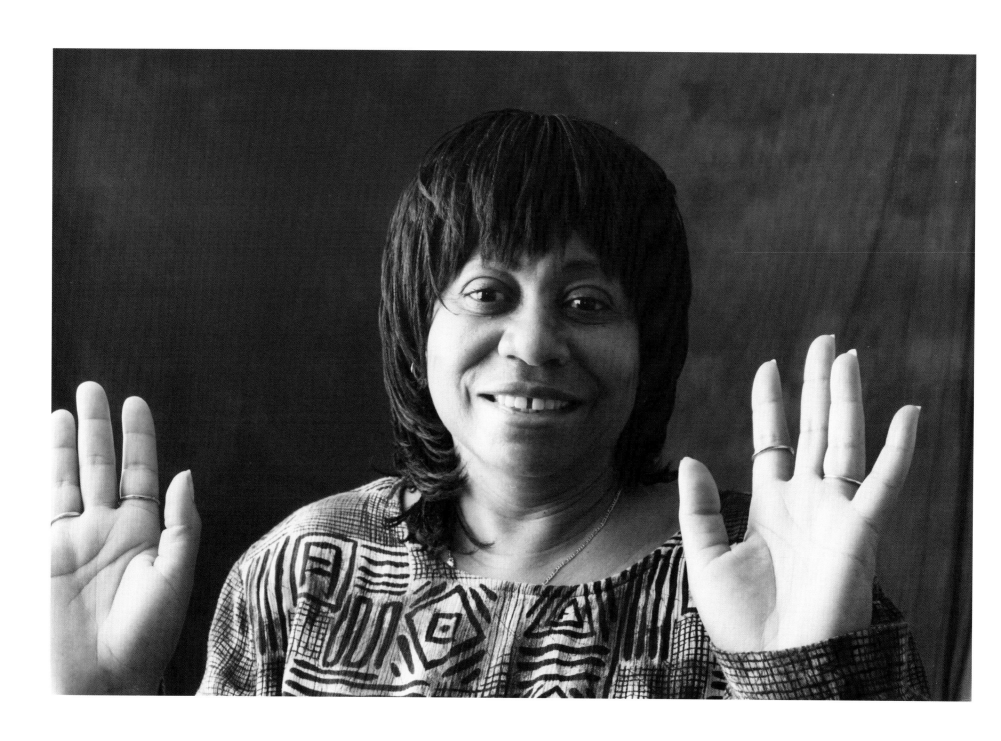

I am 58 years old, but going to be 39 on this next birthday. I had always seen how to do a self breast exam on television, but it's very different when you find a lump on your own breast.

I found a lump on my left breast and the doctors did a biopsy. I had found the lump earlier and should have had it looked at earlier. I had just ignored the lump, perhaps I wished it would go away on its own.

The doctor said it was a "fast-growing-rare form" of breast cancer. We got started with chemotherapy and my hair fell out right away. I never went in public without wearing a wig. Then, I started radiation. The doctors wanted to do six and a half weeks, but I made them stop. It was Christmas time and I wanted to be with my family.

I have an 18 year-old granddaughter that I ham helping get a start on life.
This is my job now. My children are older and on their own.

My last check-up showed another lump, now in my right breast. If it is cancer, I will not go through further treatment.

I am thankful for each day.
I am a survivor.
I am not afraid to die.
I can accept this fact.

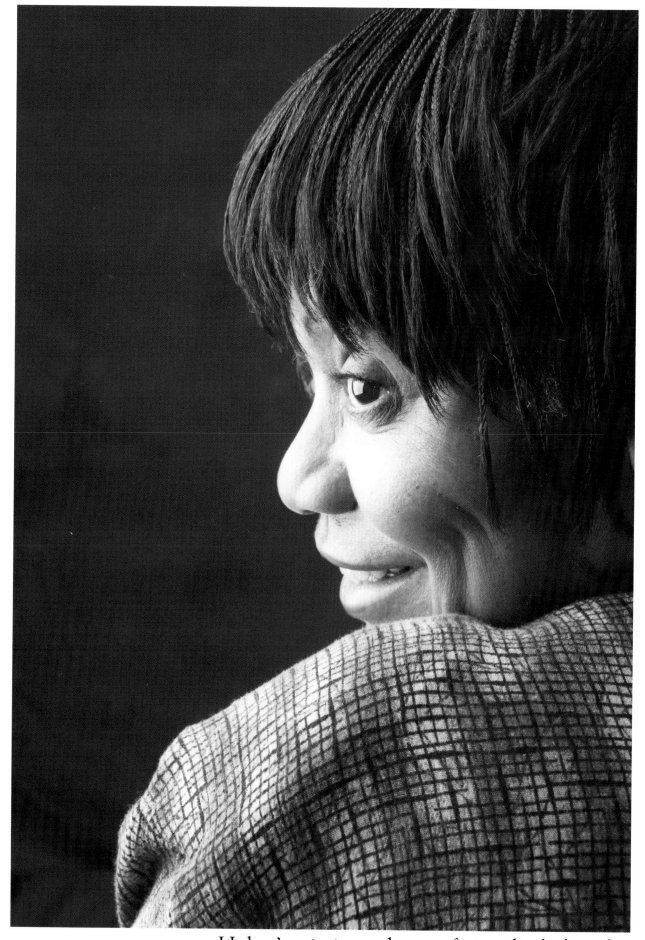

Helen's wig is made up of tiny, little braids.

I AM HAPPY TO BE ALIVE!

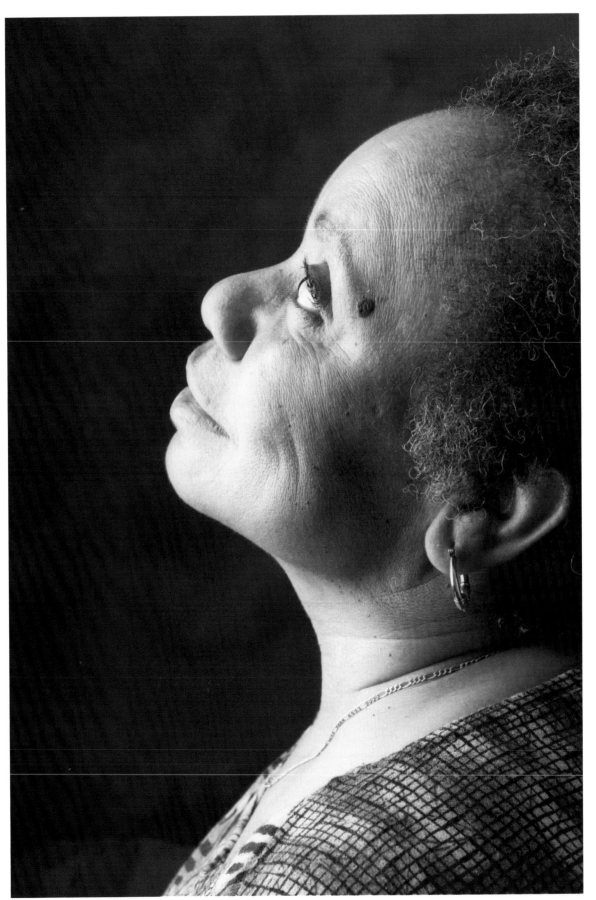

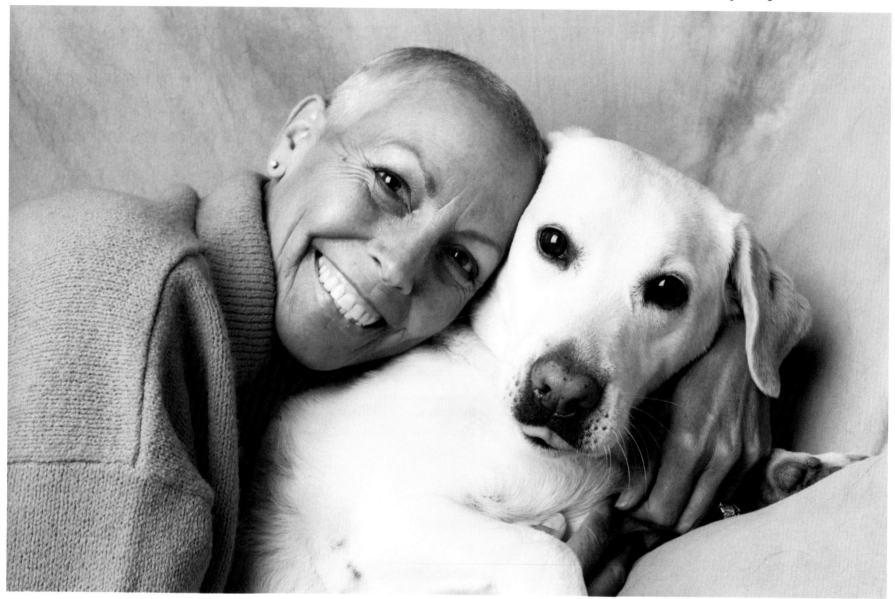

I am 53 years old and I have ovarian ccancer. I had surgery to remove both ovaries, my uterus and six inches of my intestines. After surgery I lost 53 pounds. I lost a sister to the same disease when she was only 37 years old. Her husband died 18 months later from a broken heart. My cancer has been hardest on my mom Dottie because we are best friends. I am not scared. I definately embrace life. My mom gave me her china set that she got for her 25th wedding anniversary. I had picked out the color and style. Now I use it as everyday dishes.

I like being bald. I still feel beautiful.

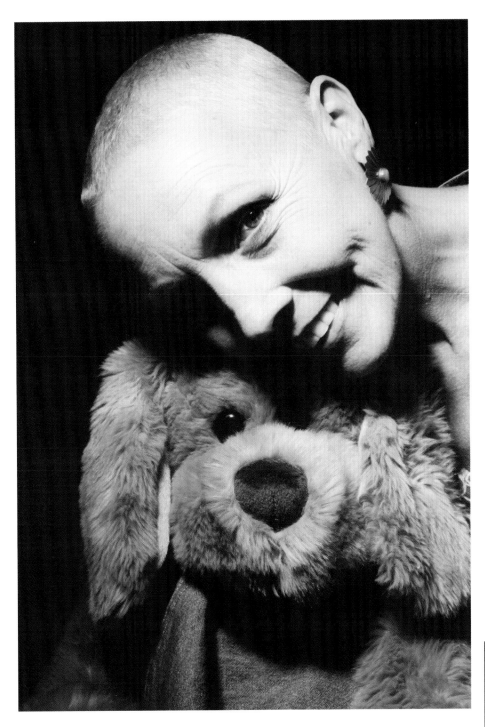

One time when I was in the hospital,
I became very, very depressed. I was
alone--without my husband, dog or
family. I kept calling my sister Linda and
she finally asked, "Do you want me to
come to the hospital?"
I told her "NO," only because I felt badly.
At 10:30 p.m., Linda showed up in my
room. Her hands were behind her back
and she was smiling. She said,
"I brought you a friend
and his name is Buddy." She held out
a fuzzy stuffed dog and put
him in my bed to keep me company.

Since then, Buddy has become my
companion anytime that I can't bring
my dog Chloe to the hospital or
anywhere else. He comes with me to
get chemotherapy; all the nurses know
him by name. When someone calls
the nurse's station asking to see if
I am there, the nurse says,
"Yup, she and Buddy are here."

Deborah & Buddy

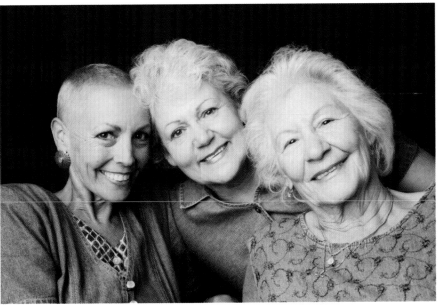

Deborah-Linda-Dottie

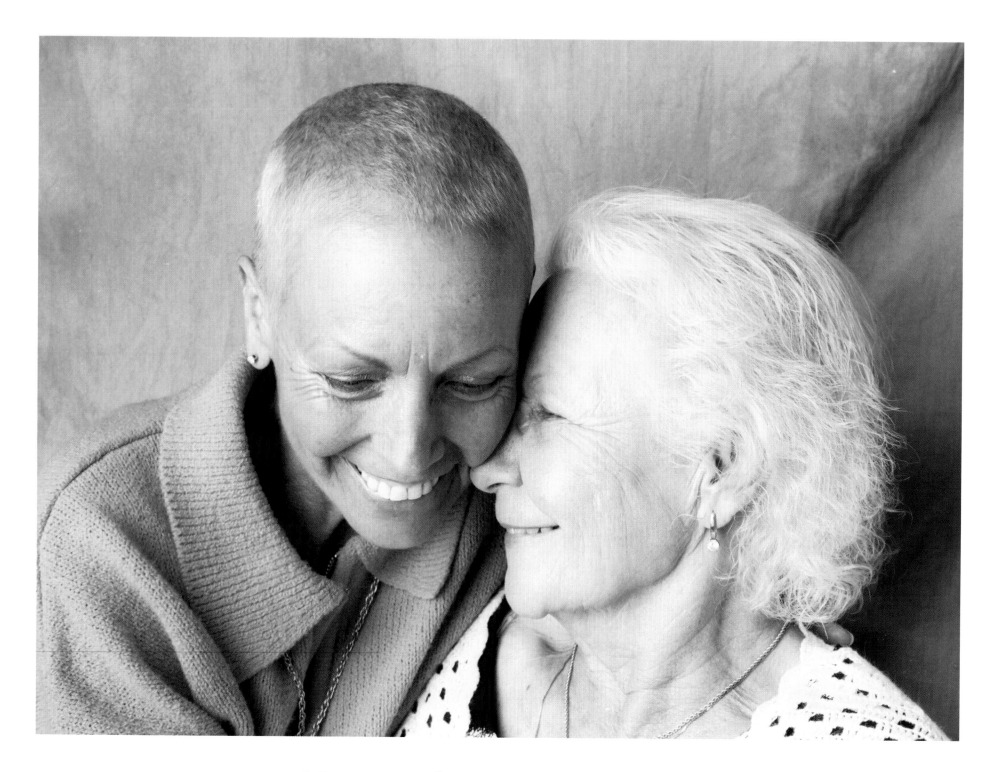

My mom is my best friend!

"There is no psychiatrist in the world like a puppy licking your face." Ben Williams

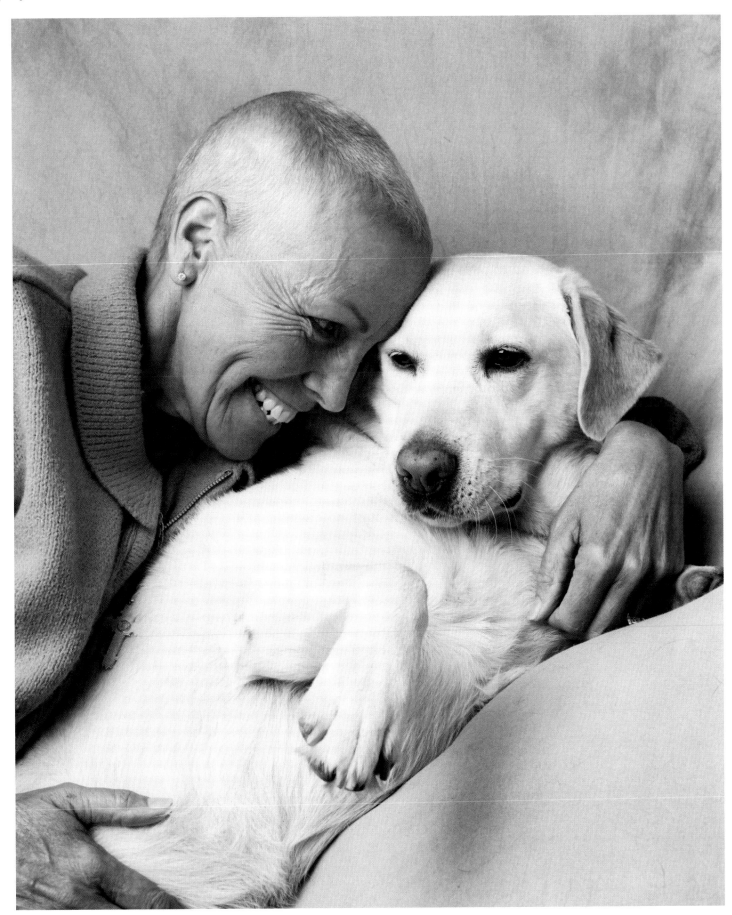

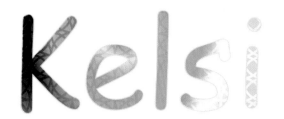

Kelsi

Goddess of...
Ambition, Tennis and Creative Writing

When I was 12 years old, I was diagnosed with Non Hodgkin's Lymphoma. I had been in Iowa and the doctor thought that I had double pneumonia. I was just about to start Junior high. I had a biopsy under my arm and neck. That's how I was diagnosed.

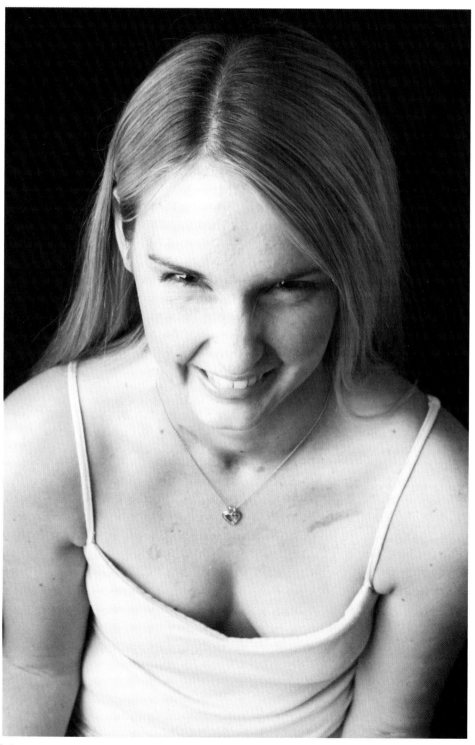

I was admitted to the hospital for four weeks for testing & testing & testing!
I remember the doctor coming to my room and I was watching TV and felt like he was interrupting me. He said, "You have a tumor in your chest." I had heard of tumors, so I asked, "Can it be removed? Am I going to die?"

My dad told me that the treatment would cause my hair to fall out. I had to stay in the hospital for the chemotherapy. My friend Miranda came to the hospital; we cried together. My treatment lasted one and half years. Every week I had to get blood tests.

I tried to go to school in between chemotherapy. I had a hard time. I got addicted to Vicodin and my dad always pretended that I wasn't sick. I was bald and pale and this mean boy started calling me "Powder" or "Casper."
I will still graduate with my friends. I just have a full class-load now to catch up.

Today I partake in telethons for cancer. I play tennis and write poetry.

All of this has made
me grow up
too fast.

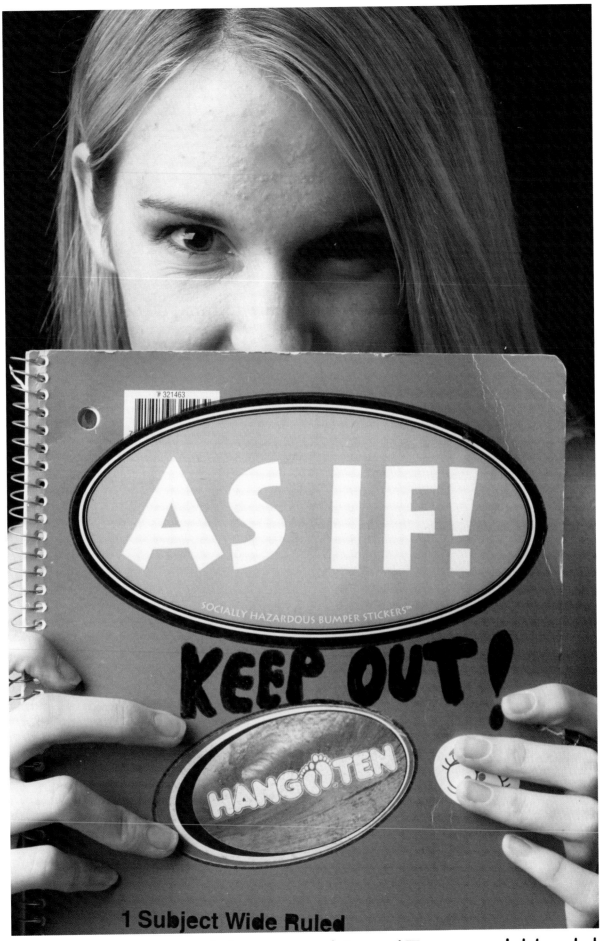

I am a 30 year old trapped in a 17 year old body!

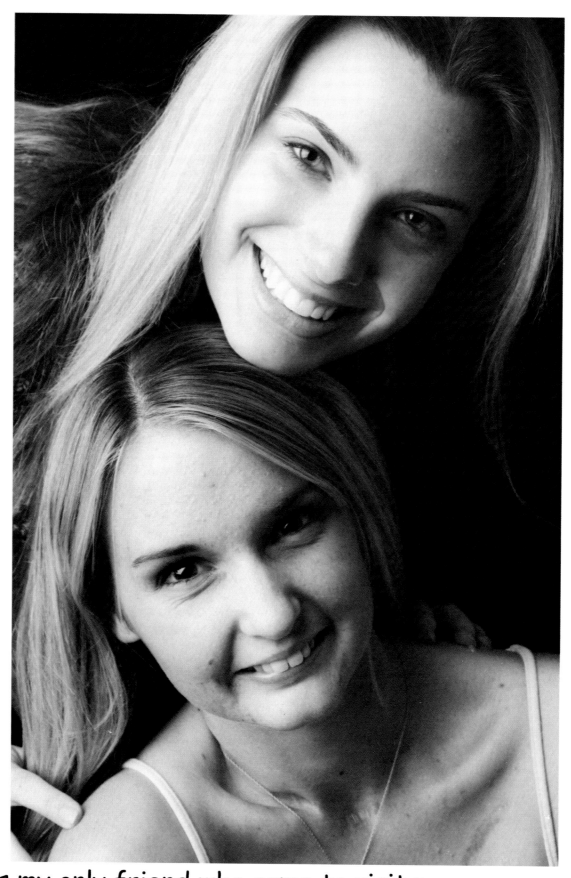

Miranda was my only friend who came to visit me
when I was in the hospital.

We have been friends since Kindergarden

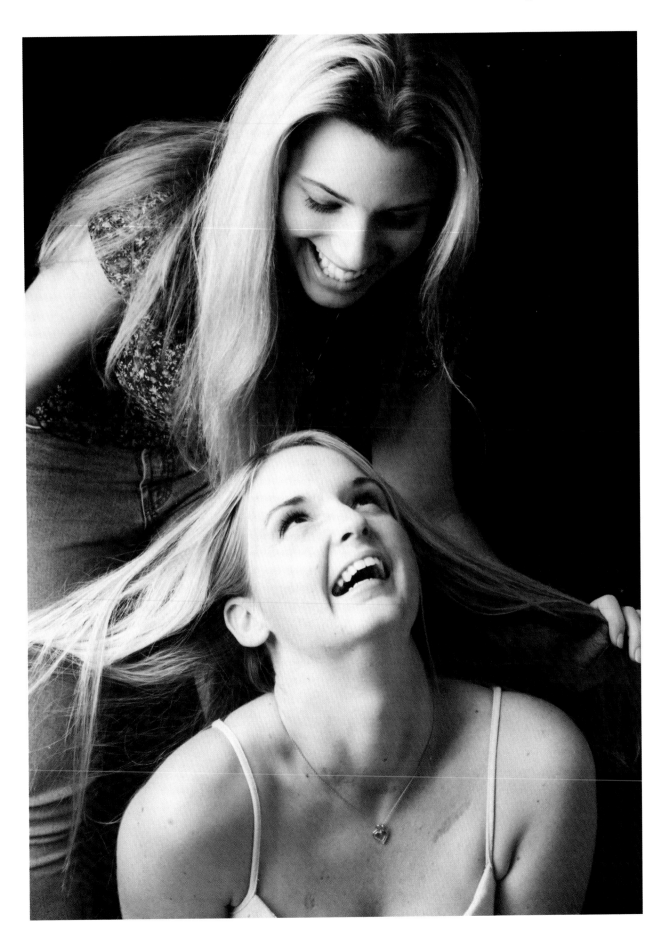

Roberta
Goddess of.. Knowledge, Endurance and Attitude

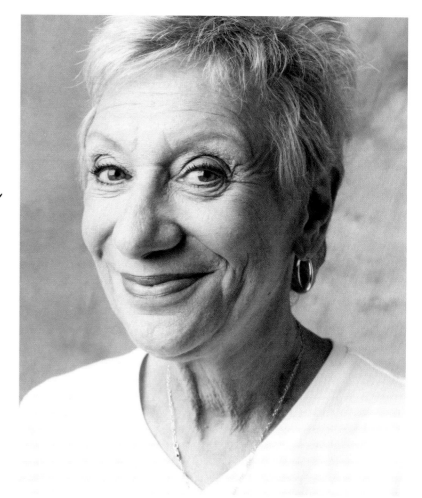

I was diagnosed with bilateral breast cancer.
To have it on both sides was a shock.
I had chemotherapy.

A few years later, the cancer came back. I had chemotherapy
again and got turned on to accupuncture.

Sammy's Grammy!

I was nauseated from chemotherapy so I tried smoking pot.
I needed it for my appetite, so I would sneak into the bathroom
and get stoned. I felt like I was 17 years old again and I felt naughty.

I joined a group of women in New York called SHARE.
The word SHARE does not stand for anything, just the literal meaning of the word.
We are a women's group that is empowering. We do walks and raise money for things.

My daughter Stace is a licensed accupuncturist and she taught me a lot about nutrition.
My son David also offered advice for healthy ways to live.

I am a grandma to Sam!

The best part about your hair falling out is, you don't have to shave your legs or tweeze your eyebrows.

My license plate says: DFWM. This stands for: "Don't Fuck With Me."
    And believe me, nobody does!

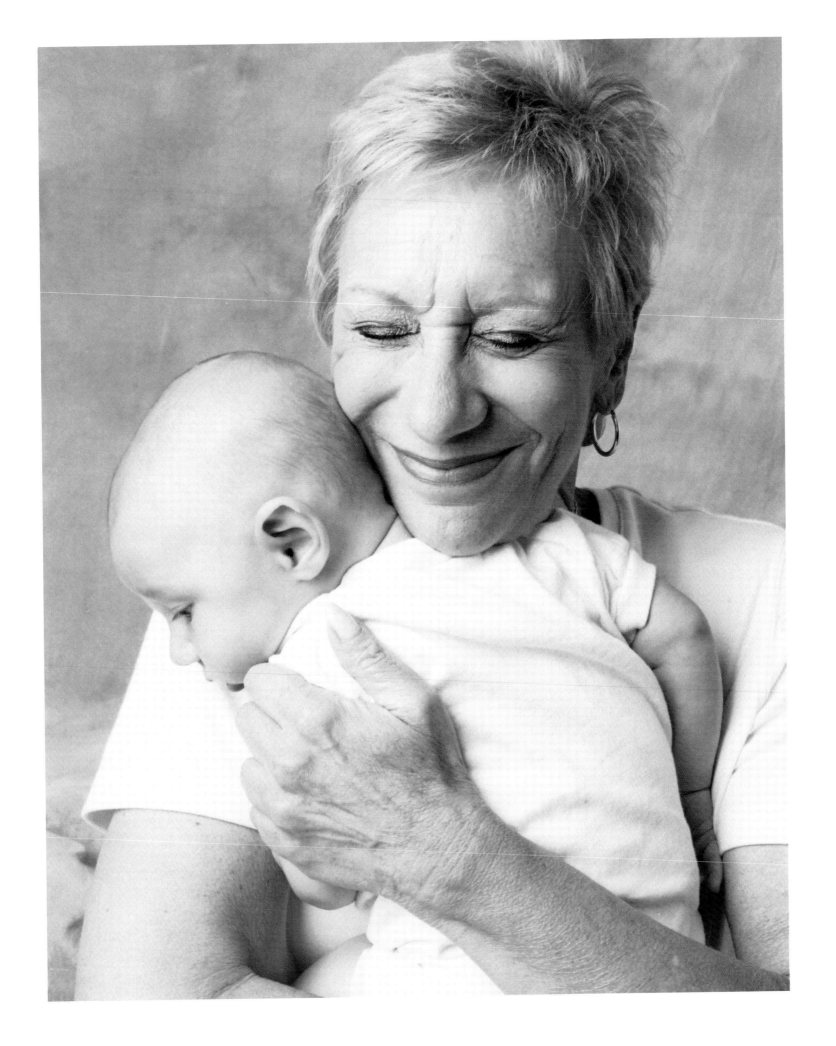

Britney

Goddess of... Giggling, Playfulness and Blonde jokes

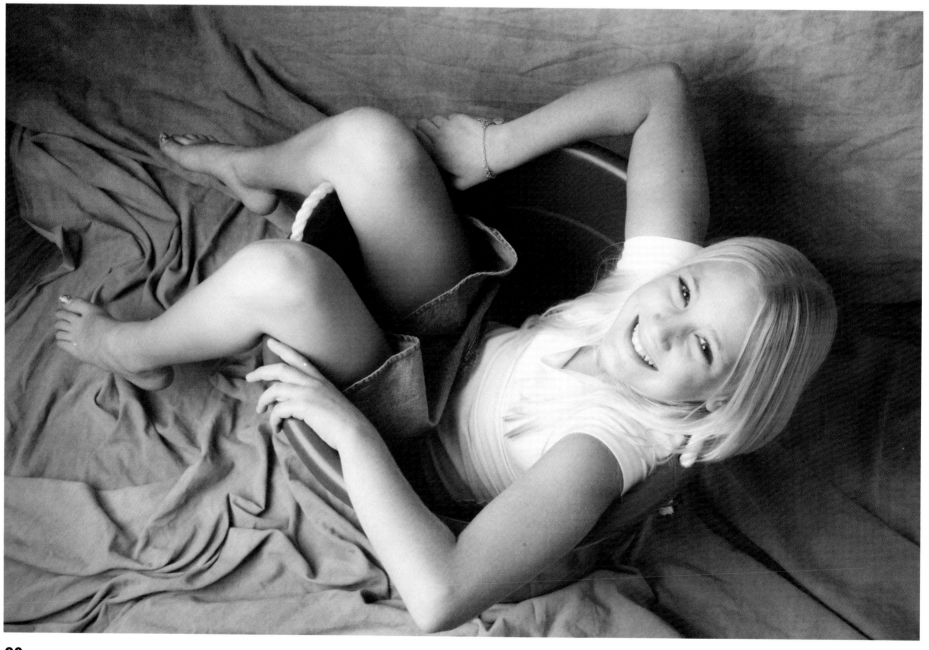

I am **12 years old.** I am a little girl with a grown ups' cancer-- It's called a **Myofibroblastic tumor.**

It started out when I could feel this huge tumor in my belly and I had a lot of pain. The doctors had not seen this kind of tumor since 1960 and it was in a grown man. I think he died?!

We knew something was wrong; I was unable to eat and all I wanted to do was sleep. I did not want to go out and play with my friends. When I would lie on my back, you could see and feel the tumors in my belly. At first, when my stomach hurt, the doctors thought I had a virus. I have had four surgeries.

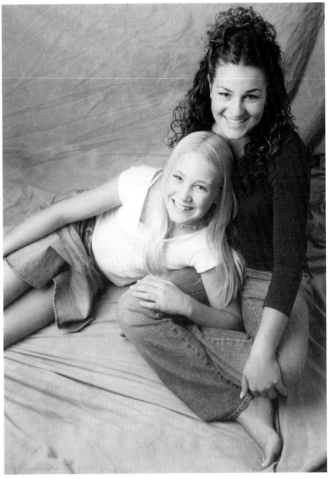

The first time the tumor was wrapped around my small and large intestines.
The second surgery the tumor was wrapped around my colon and intestines.
The third surgery the doctors tried to remove the tumor, but it was too crazy.

Six months later I ended up at the hospital called, *City of Hope*.
They tried an experimental drug called *Gleevic*.
I felt sick all the time and it did not shrink the tumor.

The doctors then decided to try chemotherapy.
Vinblastine and Methotrexate.
I started this chemotherapy 2 years ago.
The doctors really did not know if this would work.
The chemotherapy has started shrinking, calcifying
and drying up the tumor. It has turned it into a rock.

The plan is uncertain.
The doctors may want to take out the tumor,
but they really are not sure. They might try to laser it out.

I have missed most of second grade and some of third grade.
The hospitals have tutors and they helped me get to the next grade at
school. I am now in the seventh grade. My favorite subject right now is
science. I have the best teacher in the world. We don't have to disect
anything. My math teacher is neat. She had cancer on her face and has
to wear an eye patch; she likes to dress up like a pirate.

I have one sister, Megan. She just turned 18. We are very close. I tease her that she's only nice to me when I am sick. I guess we have normal sister arguments; I like to steal her clothes or go into her room when she's on the phone. I think everything is funny. I love apple pie. I know a million blonde jokes.

One time, when I was in the hospital, I was getting ready for a big surgery. The doctors wanted all my insides cleaned out, so I had to drink this nasty stuff called Golytely. It's really salty and it makes you go pooh instantly. I really did not want to drink it. I was crying. My entire family was in my hospital room and they were trying to encourge me to drink the stuff. My cousin Justin threw a dollar down and said, "You can have this if you drink it." Well, that started a family trend. The money started flying and I started drinking. I made $200.

I took some of the money and bought my sister a birthday present from the hospital gift shop. It was her birthday and I felt badly that I was having surgery on her birthday. I got her some nail polish, and a teddy bear.

I am a little girl with a grown-up cancer

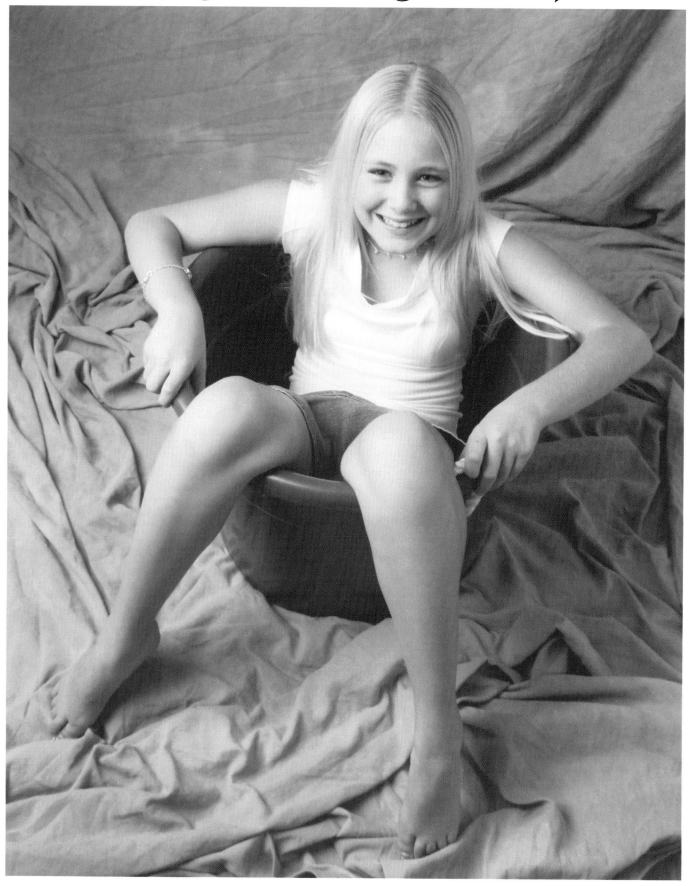

I was invited to the Ronald McDonald Camp -- the first time was in 2000. It was so cool. You eat a lot. The food is amazing. I always tell people that there are no cooks at camp, only chefs. You drive up to the mountains and take a bus to get there. You stay in a cabin with bunk beds and there are a lot of activities to do. I love to horseback ride, swim, and do arts and crafts. This year I finally got to do the **courage course tower.** You can only go to the camp until you turn 18. Then you can be a counselor, which I would like to do. The other neat thing, is that my sister can go to the camp with me. I have made a lot of friends there.

I got a wish granted by "Make a Wish Foundation"....
I got to swim with the dolphins in Hawaii.

I think I am a happy, perky person.
I don't think it's nice to make fun of other people.
I am just not like that!

I am not sure what I think about heaven.
I think more about where did we come from?
How did all the stuff on earth start? How will it end?
Those questions are what I spend more time thinking about.
I guess when two of the other patients that I have known during my hospital stays died, it felt weird. Otherwise,

I just don't think about dying.

When I grow up, I used to want to be a vet. Now I want to be a *child life specialist.* I met a bunch at UCLA and they are awesome. They are special people that are trained to make you feel happy while you are in the hospital. They talk to you about your sickness and read to you and take you on walks. They are safe. I was in the playroom with one and the doctors are not allowed to give you treaments while you are with them. NO poking or medicine. Most of them are funny. One of them, I think he was studying to be a doctor, he always made me laugh. He would wear glasses with slinky eyes. I had a bellyache from laughing at him.

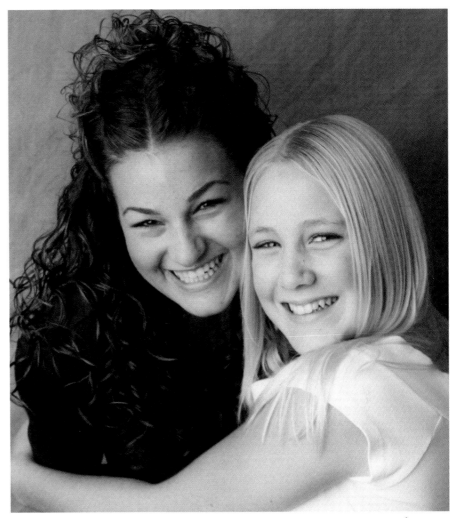

Megan & Britney

My family is what gets me through all the scary stuff. I used to think my mom did not love me when she would have to hold me down to get a shot or an IV. I understand that she was just trying to make me better.

I think that I have broken all the science rules with this tumor. I was told that I would die. I was told I would never grow, and I am already 4'11". I am almost as tall as my sister. This is funny.

I have a big scar down my tummy. When the surgical staples were there, it looked like a railroad track. I used to take puffy-pens and draw on my belly. I would make flowers or other designs.

I used to have a dog named Jasmine. She was my friend. She helped me heal emotionally because she would always just be next to me when I would not feel good. She died of cancer; I think that's weird.

In the hospital, dogs would come to visit. One time a big, snowball like dog slept on my bed. He wouldn't leave to go to the next patient. It was cute.

Sometimes I just don't feel well. I want to sleep all day. I won't want to do homework or play with my friends. I like to watch movies during these times. I guess that's just part of having cancer. I feel good most of the time. Maybe I'll write a book about my life. In some ways, I feel like I have grown up fast, but then again, I know I am just a kid. I don't get discouraged. My family and I talk a lot about being sick. I did a show-and-tell school project in the fifth grade about my cancer. The nurse came to my school. That was how I broke the news to my school about what was going on with me. I feel lucky that there are no secrets. I know that I have had a different life than a lot of other girls, but I just want to be treated the same.

Cindy
Goddess of...
Love,
Inner energy
and
Creativity

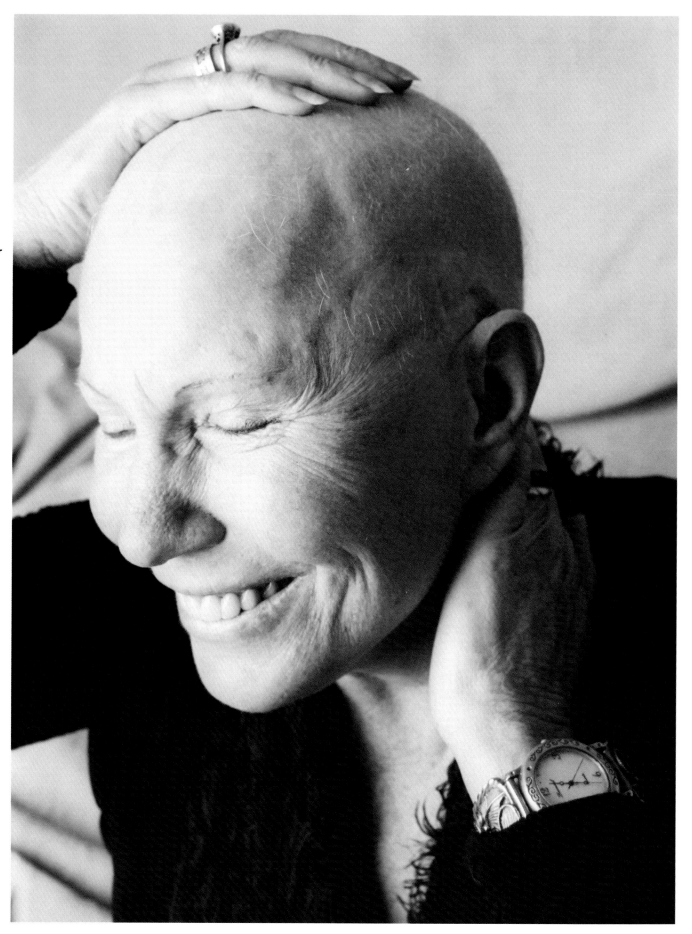

I was raised in the Outback of Australia. Then I lived in London, and then New York.
I never tell my age. Today, I have made a life in the states, but keep my citizenship in Australia.
We grew up with the idea that you don't go to doctors. I was always healthy, I figured your body
could heal itself with exercise, attitude and food. I am not a good advocate regarding mammograms
and pap-smears, because I have never had them.

In 1995 I was in a car accident. I went blind in my left eye and I was told I would never walk again.
I healed. The past three years were most content; life was good. I sold my house and simplified
my life. I know about Love, Buddha, and minimal belongings.
Eat right, love, and be creative.

Then, I found this lump in my breast. I was pissed off that I had to seek traditional medicine.
Originally I ignored the lump, as I had one in 1995 and it went away. The lump just continued to
grow. It was the size of a golf ball and was located high up on my breast. I looked like I had three
breasts. It was considered an invasive tumor and had spread to my lung. It's counterproductive
to think, "Where did this come from?" That's a waste of energy. Next month I'll have surgery;
a radical mastectomy.

The doctor started chemotherapy on me immediately. Since this is a fast growing tumor--there is no
time to think. Chemotherapy made my hair fall out in bits and pieces, not clumps like I had
imagined. It's weird to be bald. I always had nice hair. It was part of my persona.
I look in the mirror and feel like, "Who is that?" I don't have hair anywhere, including my eyebrows
and eyelashes. It is insulting to have to draw in my eyebrows with a make-up pencil.

I get accupuncture after chemotherapy to help with nausea. It's working, because I have not
had any nausea. I do not know if I will have reconstruction. I cannot think that far ahead right now.
I have seen other women who have had reconstruction and they look beautiful. Who knows?!

One step at a time!

You have to have your priorities straight!

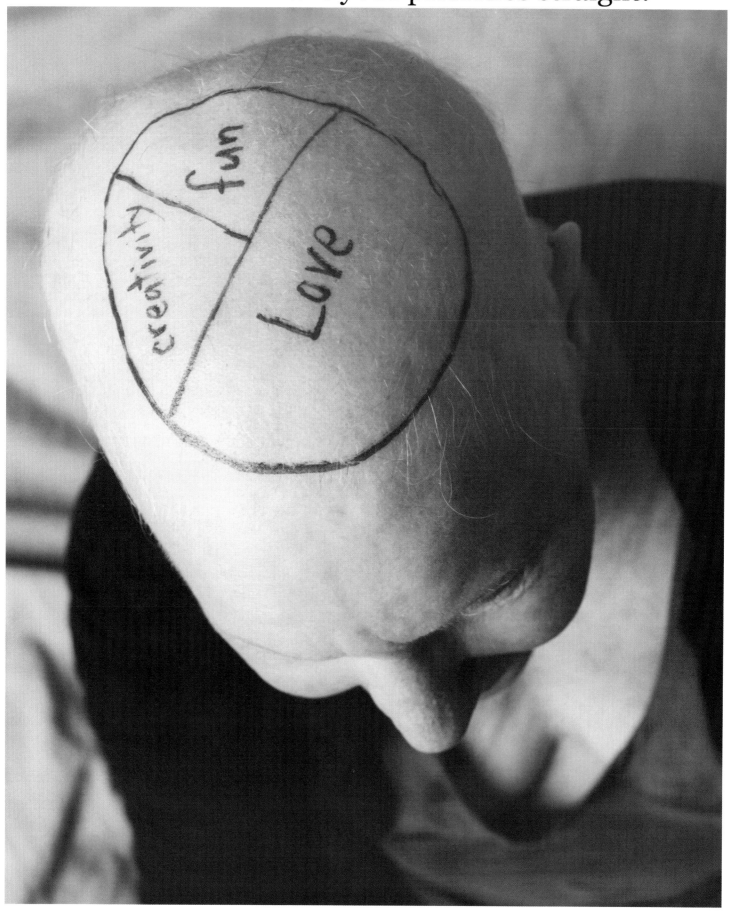

I practice Qigong. It's a 5,000-year-old Chinese healing discipline.
It teaches you to bring the chi (energy) into your body.
We are all a field of energy. We are all part of each other.

This life is part of a bigger picture. I have learned a lot about love and receiving love.
I used to be so stoic...I thought I could do everything by myself. I was married and have been
in relationships---perhaps I was more superficial then.

I love people.

I love being creative and having fun.
I cry sometimes in happiness. People are so capable of giving so much love,
I never knew that before all of this. Since I have had cancer, new people have come into my life.
There are these two women who have become my friends and they are wonderful--Rose and Karen.
After my chemotherapy treatments they take care of me.
They never get tired of waiting on me and feeding me *Jell-O*. I'm so lucky to know them!

I used to try to fix and change people. What a relief that I don't feel that way anymore.
I don't give advice; I just like to listen. I don't offer an opinion. What do I know?
I cannot fix them. I can only fix me. My path may not be healed---that's okay. I am not scared to die.
Albert Einstein said that we are all made of the same stuff. I agree with that. When we leave the body,
we enter another dimension. I have had a good life. Good vs. Bad...nothing is one or another.
I am no better (or worse off) than anyone else. You just go down the path. It's not about destination.
Cancer is not about surgery or healing. It's just a course and path. I don't chase down my test results.
I refuse to be categorized as a cancer patient. I am a person. I don't like to tell my age, marital status,
or job. In a past life, maybe I had five children? This life I do not have any.

I now wear sillier clothes than ever.

I had been so casual. I love wild scarves,
skirts, and I show off my legs. I had been writing a book about my life, and am about 30 pages
away from completion. I will write again...I am temporarily distracted at the moment.
All I want is to be healthy, have a vegetable garden, soul-mate and a dog or cat.

Right now...I am having fun. I am now very impulsive.

I went into the ocean with my clothes on when I was at the beach with my friend. I did not care.
The ocean felt great and made me laugh. That felt so good. I would not have done that before all of this.
People probably thought we were nuts, but I do not care!

Goddess of... Sunni
Cheer, Medication and a Personal experience

I have been a registered nurse for 28 years.
I have been an oncology nurse for nine years.
It seems ironic that I was diagnosed with cervical cancer.
Compared to most of my patients, I got off easy.
I had surgery and did not have to endure chemotherapy
or radiation. I was very business-like throughout the whole
treatment.

I am upbeat naturally.
It is not depressing to care for patients that have cancer.
There are times when someone is sad or hurting and this
does affect me.

I work with four Oncologists in a private practice.
I am in charge of the "outpatient" treatments. I have my own,
fairly large room that is part of the doctor's office. It has been
nicknamed, "Sunni's Cocktail Lounge." There are about eight
lazy-boy-type chairs set up in a semi circle with IV poles right
next to them. My patients come for their medications throughout
the day. Some are there for a quick shot and some stay for
hours. Some patients come once a week and some come everyday.
They seem get to know each other really well, especially those
that are on the same schedule or receiving similar drugs or have the
similar type of cancer.

I have pictures of our patients on the walls, poems they wrote
that I have framed and many stuffed animals all over the place.
I have tried to make the room less sterile and more warm and
home-like.

I do have my favorite patients--but my relationship with
all my patients goes beyond calling them Mr or Miss So and So.
I see them as a whole person who have familes and feelings.

I give them chemotherapy and other medications to help
save their lives. I give all kinds of drugs--ones that calm people
down, relieve nausea, prevent an allergic reaction and some
that help rebuild the white or red blood cells. I feel like I have such power and
control with these medications. What a contradiction that I too got cancer. The world is a a funny place.

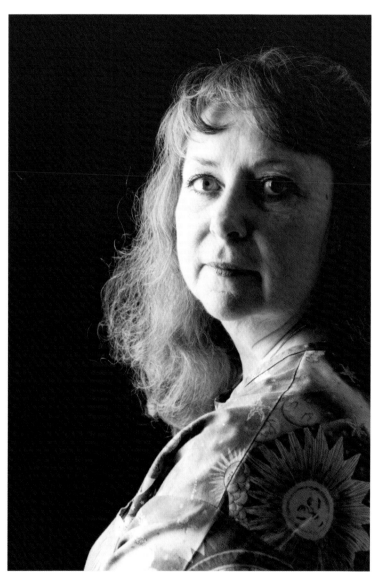

Sunni likes to wear nursing scrubs that are decorated with suns

"As an Oncology nurse I don't think of myself as an angel, just a constant in my patient's changing lives."

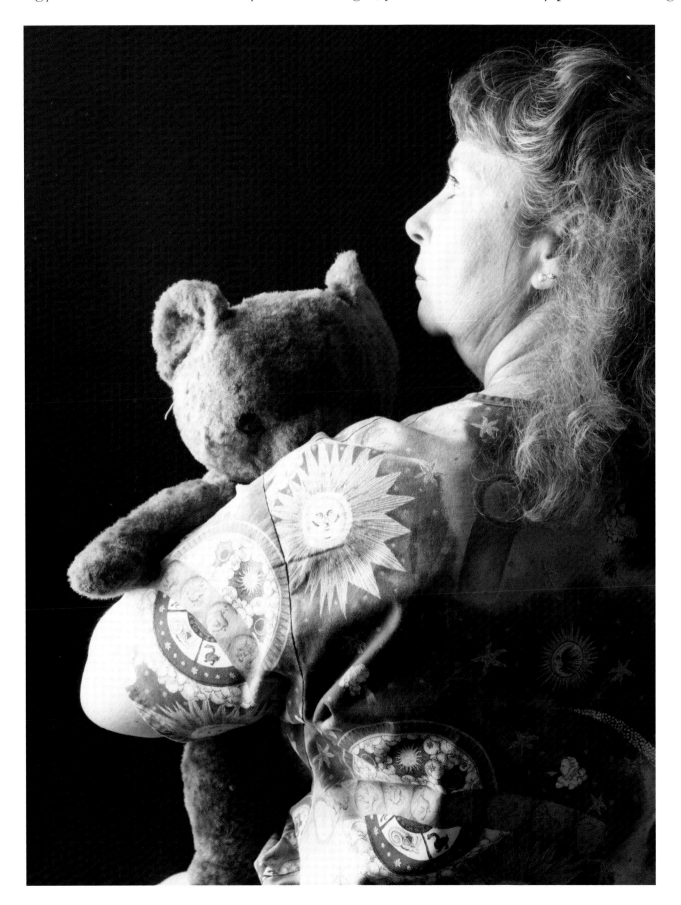

Lesley
Goddess of... Positive Thinking, Defiance and Acceptance!

In March, I was diagnosed with breast cancer. At the time, the doctors did a lumpectomy. Three years later, in November, I was diagnosed with bilateral breast cancer. The cancer had spread to my liver. In January, I underwent a double mastectomy. I refused to have reconstuctive surgery then and continue to refuse now. I have endured several rounds of chemotherapy.

In June, I was diagnosed with a tumor on my lung. The tumor grew one centimeter a month. The doctors removed the tumor and part of my lung (called a Thoracotomy).

I received Herceptin every three weeks, I will get this forever. I still have to have yearly scans and monitor my liver. I am very involved in a breast cancer support group. We meet once a month and have breakfast and chat. We really help each other out, if some one needs to cry, we listen. If someone needs to move to another home, we are there for that too.

My doctor said to me, 'Go out and do the things you want to do.' I actually listened to him. I bought my dream car (a Miata, then a Corvette). I saw the Green Bay Packers play. I went to Europe on a cruise and visited Egypt too.

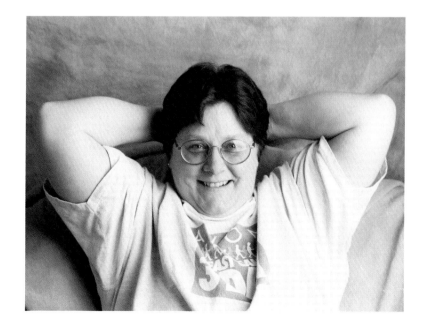

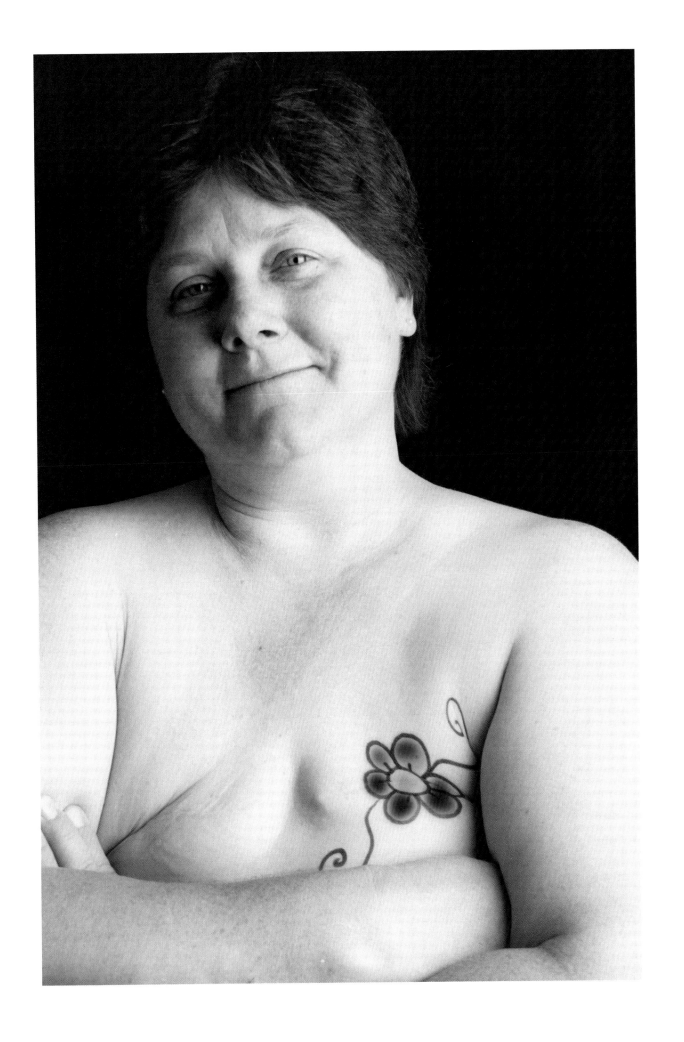

The Ventura County Star Newspaper Article
"FIGHTING FOR LIFE ON A DAILY BASIS"

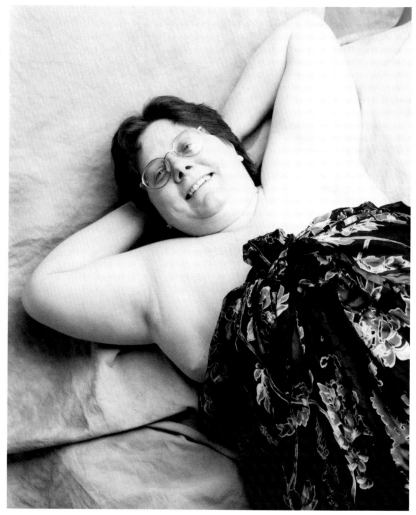

"...45 year old accountant...diagnosed with breast cancer 1996...[She had a] double mastectomy in January 2000. The cancer spread to her lungs, and she lost two thirds of her right lung a few months later...she is lively and full of personality...seemingly too chipper for a cancer patient. But she pointed out that she's had it for six years and has gone through all the emotions already. Adding that, 'I've always been really independent and obnoxious.'

'...From then on, every day has been the best day I could make it....Attitude is 99 percent of how you get by.'

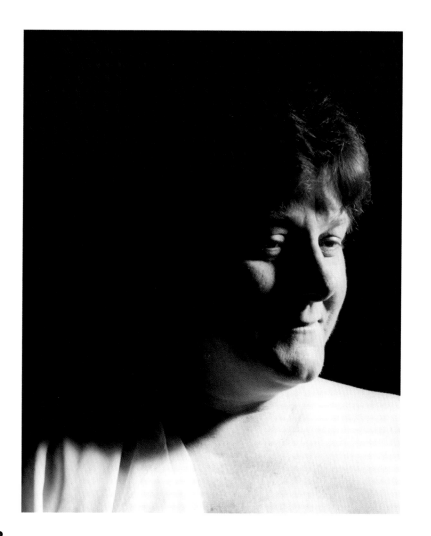

"I've got cancer, but cancer does not have me!"

"Reflection..."

This what I call these pictures.
I look at what is or isn't there. After I had the mastectomy, I thought I would have just two lines, not what I have. I am comfortable to show off my scars, they just look differently than I had expected.

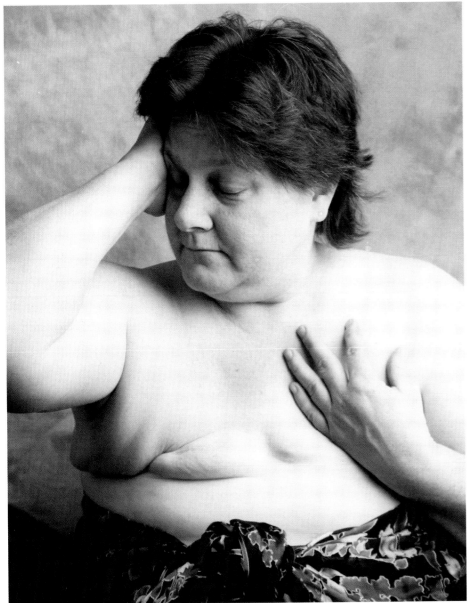

Cancer is a strange gift.
Knowing your life could end at
   any time.
I now have insight.
   Most people don't have this.

Goddess of... Kiley
Generosity, Singing and Not caring what other people think!

I am 33 years old and my passion is singing.

I was diagnosed with bilateral Dysgerminoma, an ovarian cancer in December 2001.
I had been going to the same Obstetric/Gynecologist for 12 years. Nobody had any idea what was going on. I'd been having severe abdominal pain. It got so bad, that I had to the emergency room three times; still without a diagnosis.
Then I got a false-postive pregnancy test. Upon the ultrasound, the doctors discovered I had what turned out to be cancer.

I had surgery to remove the right ovary and part of the left ovary. The official name: Salpingo-Oophorectomy.
I opted to save the left ovary because I really want to have children.
After surgery the chemical warfare began.
I had three rounds of chemotherapy, five days a week, six hours a day. bi-weekly with two days between.
I got SO nauseated and I tried all the prescribed anti-nausea medications, but they did not work.
When the Oncologist recommened, I tried smoking marijuana for my appetite. I really wasn't a pot smoker, but I surrenedered to trying it. To my surprise, it worked! The biggest surprise of smoking pot was the suppliers. Some of my most conservative friends would come over and roll me the tightest joint.

My hair has now grown back, but it's hard to shape. Surprisingly, I always felt sexy
 Here I was at 175 pounds (overweight for me) with "bad hair" and I couldn't wear shoes and I still got hit on!

I do what I want. It's too exhausting to be the fake girl. I am much happier not being "her." I am a singer. I just wrote and recorded my first solo album. I love to perform live. When people come to hear me sing, it's the greatest feeling.
I find myself singing for fundraisers, because it's not about the money. It's about standing up there and entertaining people with my gift. I love that.

I try to live my life by these words....

"Our deepest fear is not that we are inadequate. Our deepest fear is that we are powerful beyond measure. It is our light, not our darkness, that most frightens us. We ask ourselves, who am I to be brilliant, gorgeous, talented and fabulous? Actually, who are you not to be? We are each children of the creator. Playing small does not serve the world. There is nothing enlightened about shrinking so that other people won't feel insecure around us. We were born to make manifest the glory of creation that is within us. It's not just in some of us. It's in everyone!! And as we let our own light shine, we unconsciously give other people permission to do the same. As we are liberated from our own fear, our presence automatically liberates others!!" ---Nelson Mandela

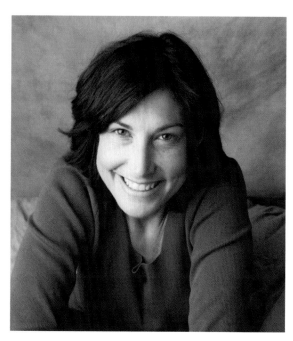

After chemotherapy, I was at an auction/fundraiser. One "item" that was up for auction was this amazing Golden Retriever puppy. Unfortunately, I became quite attached to the precious puppy-girl. People started bidding and I was not far behind. The price just got too high for my wallet. Boo! My friends were trying to buy her for me. When I realized it, I called off their ruse. She sold for $1,700!

However, an interesting thing happened. The person that won the puppy--it turned out his children were sadly allergic to her and had to give her away.

Guess who got her free of charge? ME!!!!

Her name is Bella!

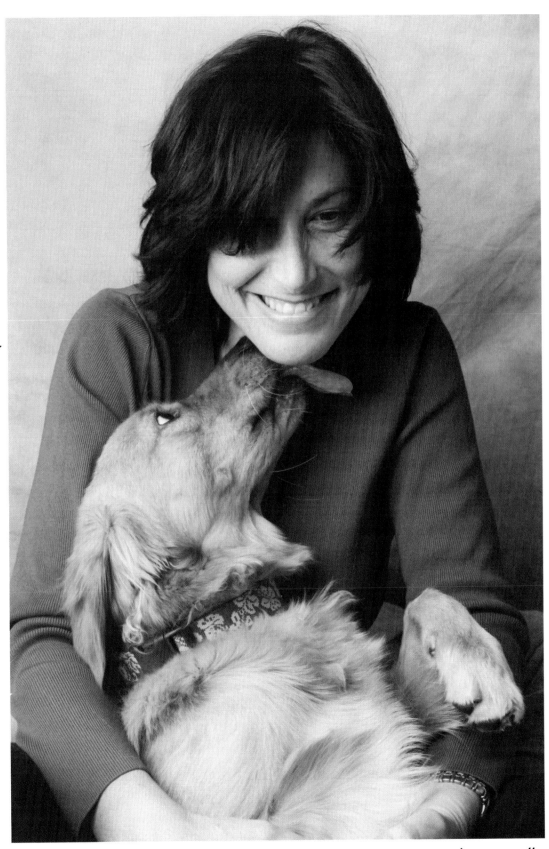

Kiley & Bella

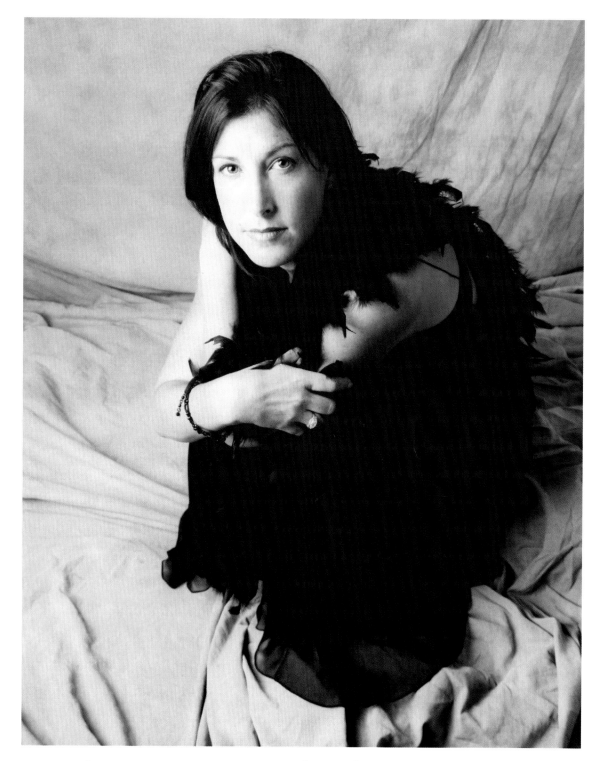

The title of my album is, "Transcending." It means to come out of something and rise above it. The songs tell my story, the process through which I have come...but a story that has passed and that I have risen or am rising above. "Stand up Tall" is my favorite song from the album.

This picture is featured on my album cover (taken by Lesley), it is part of a series of three that show me emotionally growing. Here I am, small, protected, and a little unsure. The other two pictures show me standing, singing with my arms free. The album allowed me to explore me. I have been through a lot in the past few years.

Cancer has made me stop and find my dream- singing.

Your body has good instincts!

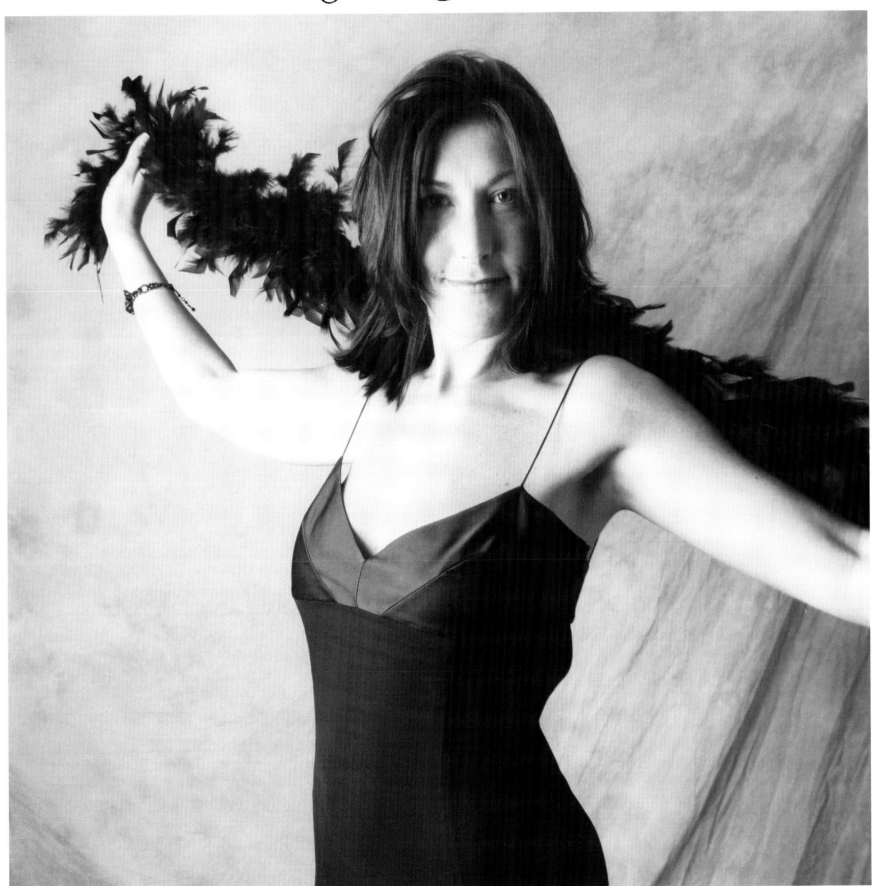

Linda

Goddess of... Believing!

On March 29th, I was diagnosed with breast
cancer. I had a double mastectomy and
four rounds of chemotherapy.

I will have reconstruction (tram flap repair) soon,
as I want my body complete.

I am 53 years old, married and have three daughters.
Their three different personalities balance me.

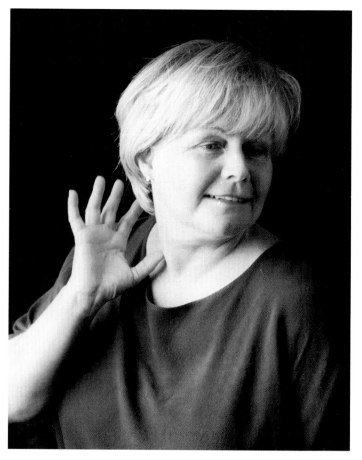

"Do you like my wig?"

A passage in an article Linda wrote titled, "On the Path to Life Insure"

"...At 39 years old, I started a fast-track life and made a career change. I started college for the first time with the goal to earn a Master's Degree as a Marriage Family Child Counselor. The stress was horrendous and took eight years to complete my education, several years to complete clinical (3,000) hours, and then pass a written and oral exam.

One month before my oral exam four little words caused my life to spin out of control. "Linda you have cancer!" The words kept coming at me; tears began streaming down my face. "Not me!" I thought. "Wasn't my mom 52 when she was diagnosed?"

As tears started pouring down my cheek, my friend put an arm around my shoulder and said, "Are you afraid of not passing?" Responding, I said, "I am not at all afraid that I won't pass...I am terrified that I won't live much longer."

**Linda said, at the point of feeling the worst in her life,
she passed her oral exam in 37 minutes!!!**

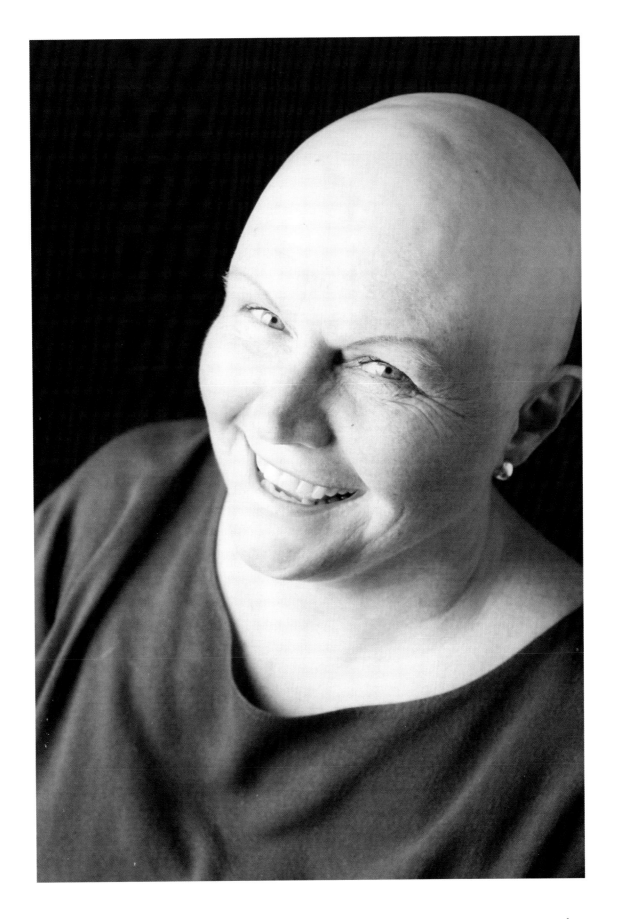

When I lost my hair (it actually flew out), it happened with 400 pieces at a time.
The wind caught the hair and sent it whirling around me in the air...   Just like a dandelion.

When Linda's daughters were asked how they felt about their mom's baldhead, they said, "It's smooth enough for a game of tic-tac-toe."

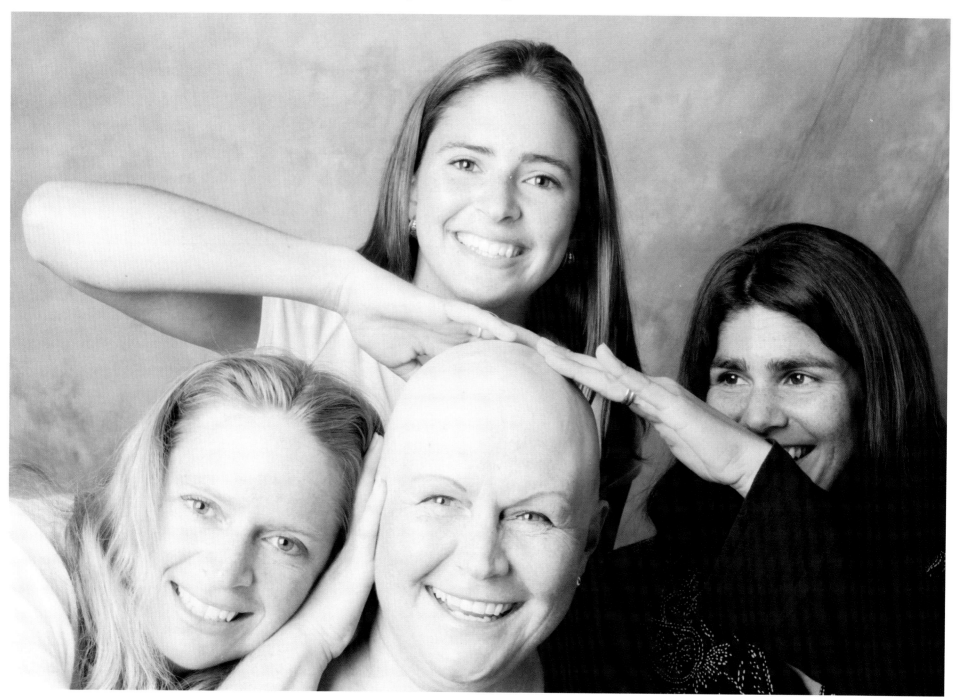

Lori, Linda, Melanie (back row) and Marci

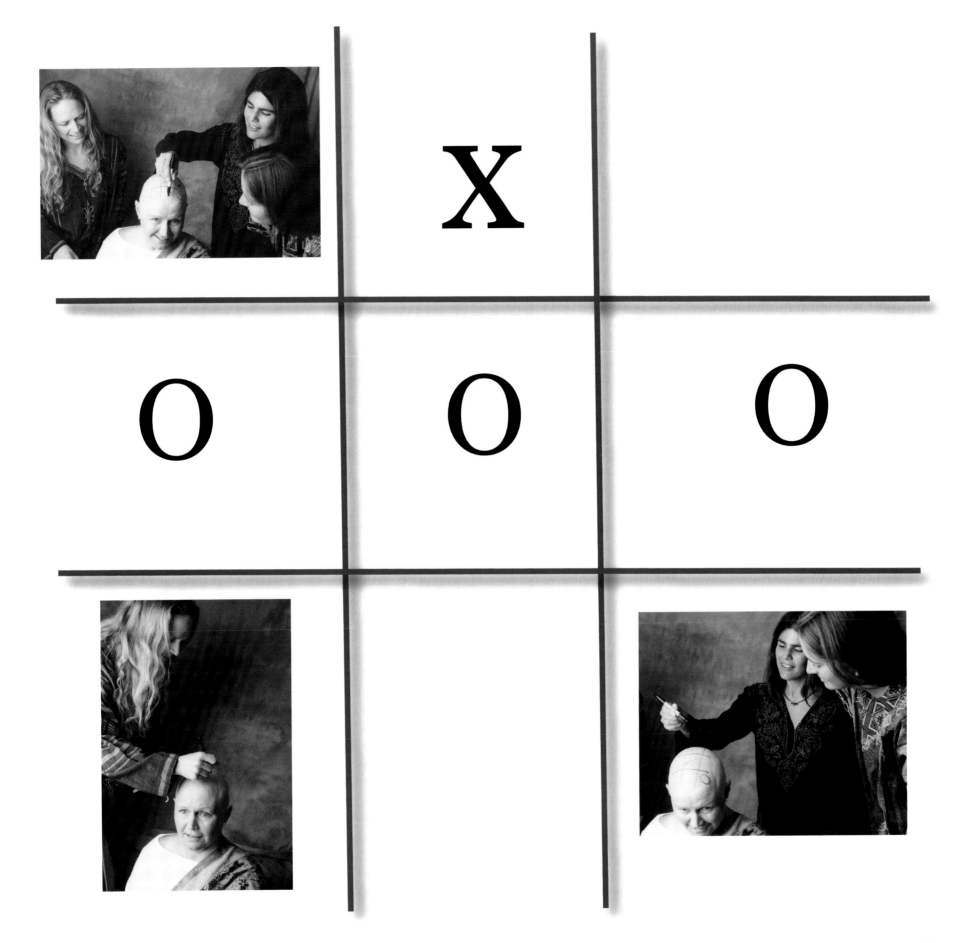

JODY

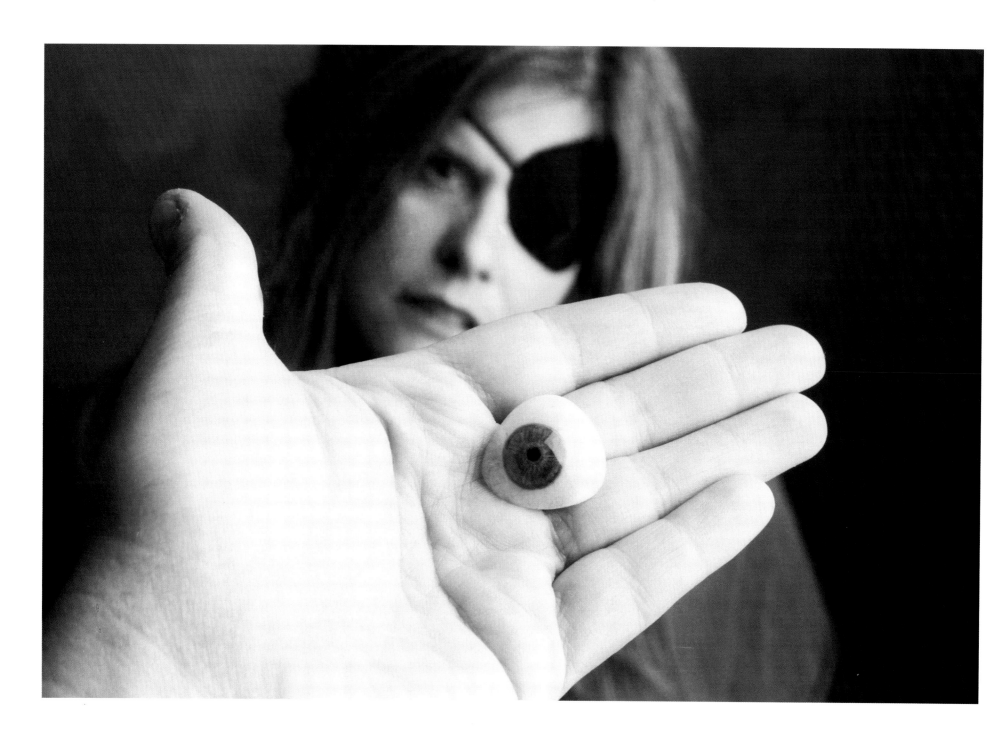

Goddess of... Laughter and A Good Heart

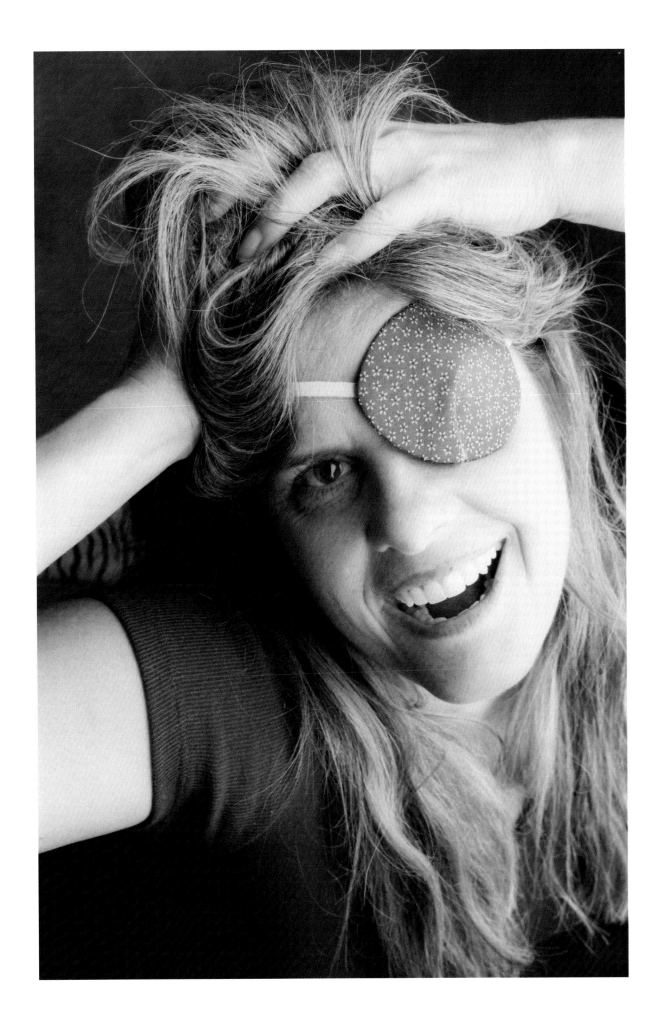

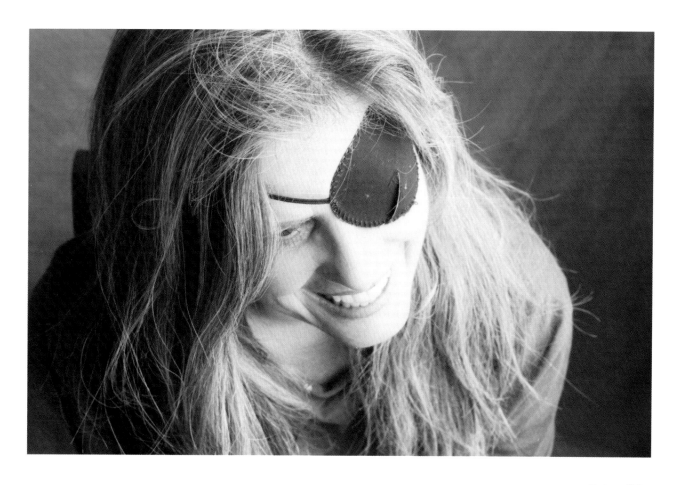

I hand-made several eye patches to match my outfits.

I have a glass eye. It's really detailed. They used red thread for the veins.

I am 40 years old and work at *Easter Seals.* I have a very rare form of **Malignant Melanoma** in my left eye. I was diagnosed in April. My vision was distorted for four days with flashes and spots. At first, the doctors tried to save my eye. I had radiation and all my eyelashes fell out.

Another doctor said that my eye should be removed. He said I had no choice. I guess you just trust that you gotta do what people say.

I am getting through this with my typical morbid sense of humor. Laughing and joking is just my personality. People have started giving me presents of Cyclops or stickers of eyeballs. The whole thing just cracks me up. Eyeballs tend to be so disgusting.

I fell in love through all of this. His name is John! Since I had to go so far a way for my treatments, we would chat excessively on the telephone. He was the calming voice on the other end of the phone line. He was so kind to me, even though the relationship was new. We have a strong connection and we are both into music. We wrote a song together.

All of this has happened very fast. I don't do much research, I find it too overwhelming. I don't know what will happen next or if the cancer is gone. **I have today. I have my love, my family & friends and my sense of humor.**

What more could a girl want?

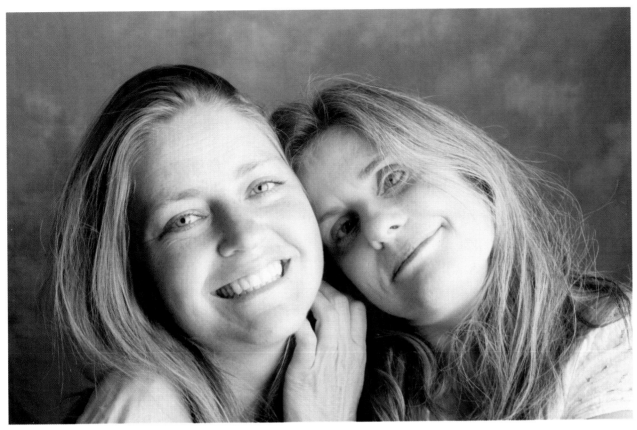

My friend Johanna is wonderful!
We swear we are long lost twins, separated at birth.
She has the same blue-colored eyes as I do.
However, she has a fleck of brown in one of her eyes.
When I had my glass eye made, I had them put the same fleck of brown in my glass eye, so we could be REAL twins!

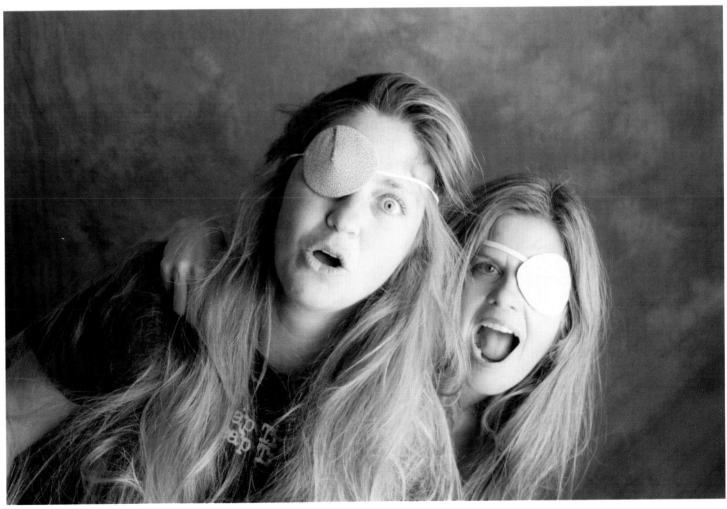

Virginia

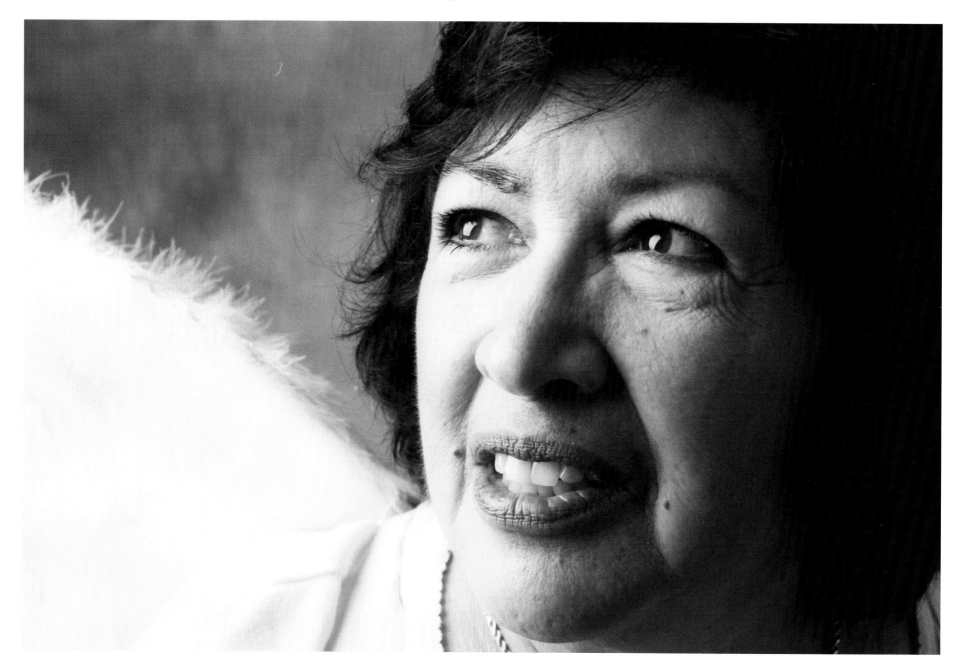

Goddess of... Personal Growth and A Sixth sense!

She arrived for our interview.
We sat at the kitchen table.
It was clear she had a story to tell.
She admitted I was the first person
she had told it to.

I have 14 guardian angels...sometimes I can feel them touching my shoulders!

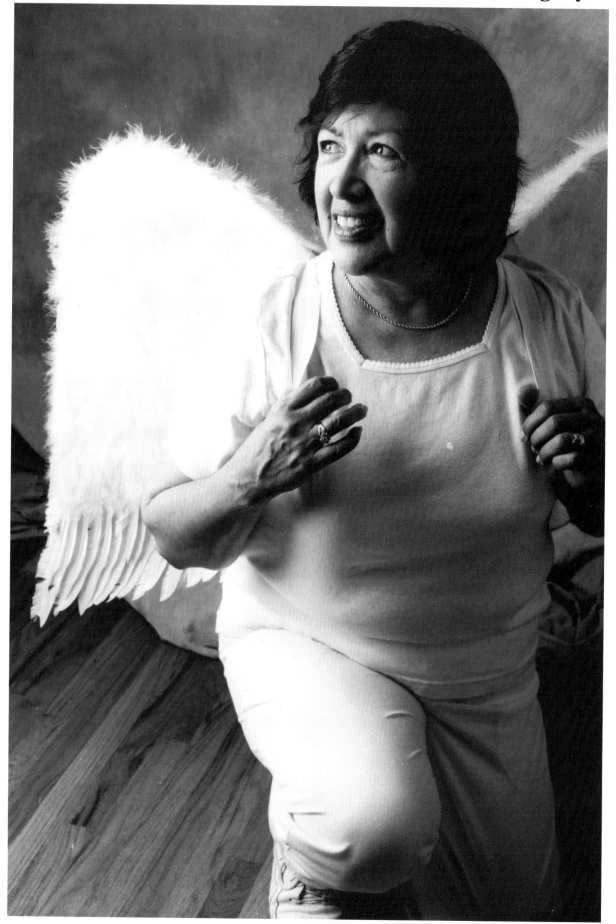

I am 62 years old, a retired clerk at the school district. I have two daughters, ages 33 and 35.
I am also a grandma.

I had been going to an accupuncturist for arthritis and told her that I was spotting and had
abdominal cramps. She suggested that I see an Obstectric/Gynecologist.

March 2002, I was diagnosed with **uterine cancer.**

The doctors did a total hysterectomy. Luckily, I did not need chemotherapy. I never looked sick.
The cancer was inside and then taken out. People had no idea what I was going through.
Nobody could tell. Some might say I got easy, but that still does not mean the experience was not
hard.

I met my husband at 14 years old. He was from a traditional home and so was I.
You did not speak unless spoken to. I realize that I have been suppressed, I love to talk.

My husband and I have had one argument, one fight that has lasted 39 years. We have
been married 41 years.

My biggest pre-cancer achievement was that when I was age 50 I ran a marathon. It took me six hours
to complete. I trained everyday. I got up to run at 5:30 am, before my husband was awake.
I did not want him to tell me not to run.

One time I was running in the dark and fell down. I felt that someone was with me, perhaps
an angel. I went to a "past life" reading and she told me that there are 14 angels guarding me.
I know one of them is my Uncle Louie who died in 1944, in the war, a premature death.

I collect angel statues and trinkets, and apparently real ones too. I think I have a sixth sense
and I am finally channeling into this.

I can't talk to anyone about how I am feeling today. I am fragmented and disconnected. I am
going to change and learn to share my emotions better.

I was submissive, but now I make each day count. I don't regret the life I had before cancer,
but now I just have a lot of catching up to do.

There are so many songs in me that have not been sung.

Gloria

Goddess of... Empathy

A few years agao, I was diagnosed with ovarian cancer.

I had Bilateral Oophorectomy -
the removal of both ovaries- with an
Omentectomy - removal of the omentum,
a layer of fat that hangs over the intestines.

I had five and half months of chemotherapy.

I am no stranger to cancer.
My husband died of cancer four years ago;

I have three children and five grandchildren....
They call me their "Nutty Grammy."

I have been a volunteer at the Sheriff's Department for two years.
I get to wear that ugly uniform and drive around in a Sheriff car.

I watch what I eat.
The portions they serve at restaurants are double the size
they need to be.
You should share your food!

Cancer has made me empathetic.
You cannot go through something like this without changing...
I feel more positive.

Also, you should never be alone. People need people!

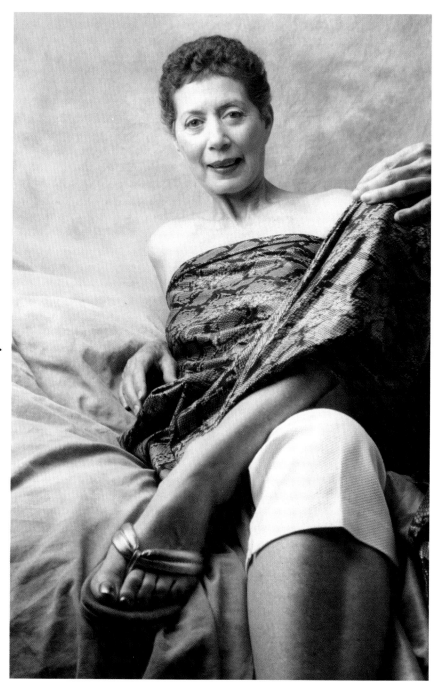

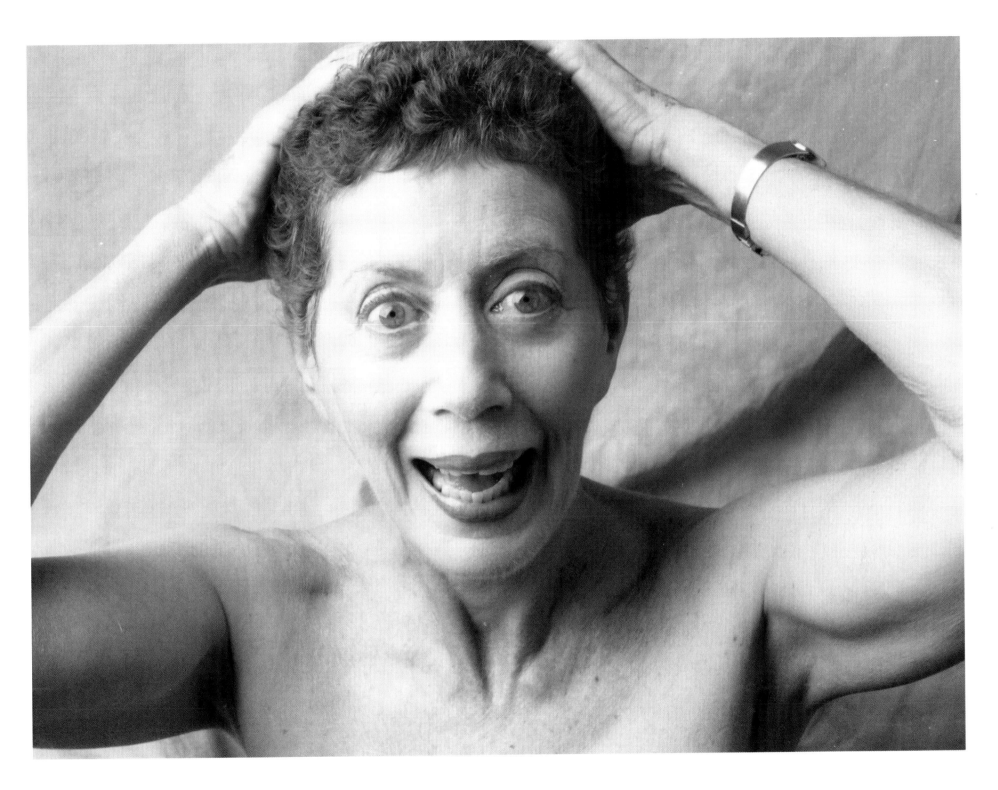

"Although the world is full of suffering, it is full also of the overcoming of it." --- Helen Keller

Linda

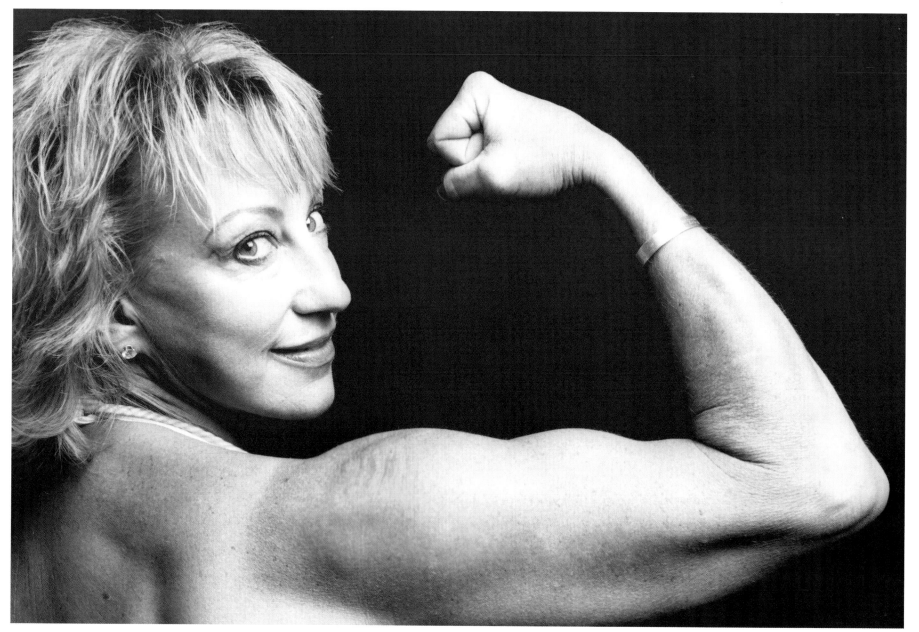

Goddess of...Might and Optimism

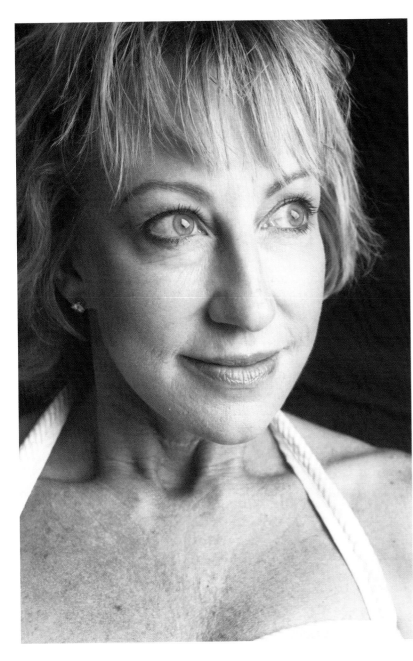

I am 44 year's old. My husband and I live on a 4,500-acre ranch.
We have 12 horses, 5 dogs, 2 cats, 23 chickens, 1 rooster, 11 ducks
and about 200 cows.

I was scheduled for a routine hysterectomy for fibroids. The surgery
was typical, not a big deal.

After the hysterectomy, I rested and sat on the couch for three days.
Then, I got up and started to refurbish the guest house that we have
on our ranch. I do not sit still well.

Five days after surgery they found cancer.
Now I was to follow the protocol for aggressive cancer.
I was to receive chemotherapy for 9 months
The pathology showed, in the centniner of the benign fibroid,
a highly aggressive form of cancer.

Leiomyosarcoma

I had a severe allergic reaction to one of the chemo-agents called Daxol.
My blood pressure dropped to 50/32. I looked at my husband and
said, "I am slipping away." The doctors reacted quickly and pumped
me full of liquids and stuff to bring my blood pressure back up.
Needless to say, they removed that medication from my
treatment regimen.

I lost most of my hair.
I was more concerned about my eyebrows.
That's your face-- your expression.

Each chemotherapy treatment, I became a little weaker and more tired
because it builds up in your system. By the seventh month,
I was SICK. I functioned by taking anti-nausea medications.
I would get home from my treatments and go out and feed the cows.
I was not going to let this get to me.

I am told that I am a miracle. I dodged the bullet.

I stayed optimistic the whole time. If the cancer returns, it will be in my lungs or liver. It will not return!

My husband Bud was absolutely amazing (he is a retired vetrinarian). He was there for everything.
During these times, you will see people's true colors.

I was always the person to help people out. When I got sick, my friends said to me, "It's now our turn to be there for you."

I do Pilates four days a week;
I feel radiant, confident and strong!

I glow of life.

I want to spread joy around the world. That is my mission. I am the light for other people.

I have a huge circle of friends, including many that I have known since high school.

I consider that I am enlightened. You can never go back, your emotions are a choice.

You should never ask, "Why me?" There is a reason. To ask is to waste time.

Just discover why. People need to embrace their calling; connect with others.

When you die, those that knew you have a piece of you in them. If you die young,

then your journey was to provide your light onto others' hearts.

What I read in pamphlets about fibroids pisses me off.

Women need to understand that fibroids can become cancerous. It happened to me.

Nine years ago there was a fibroid in my uterus that broke through the uterine wall.

The doctors removed that fibroid, but left the other one in there and that sucker is the one that

became a cancer ball.

Women **need** to know the truth!

I love being a woman. I am physically strong. I love wearing pink.
I can endure. I am sensitive. I am feminine. I am healthy.

I find fun in everything.

I am an artist; I like to draw and paint.

My newest hobby is soldering metal into beautiful jewelry

I like to take pictures and make a solder frame around them and string it onto a necklace with pretty beads.

I have done great. I feel so lucky.

People go through their whole lives and never know how many people love them. I am happy to know this.

Having cancer is part of my life, part of my journey. It's who I needed to become. I understand this now.

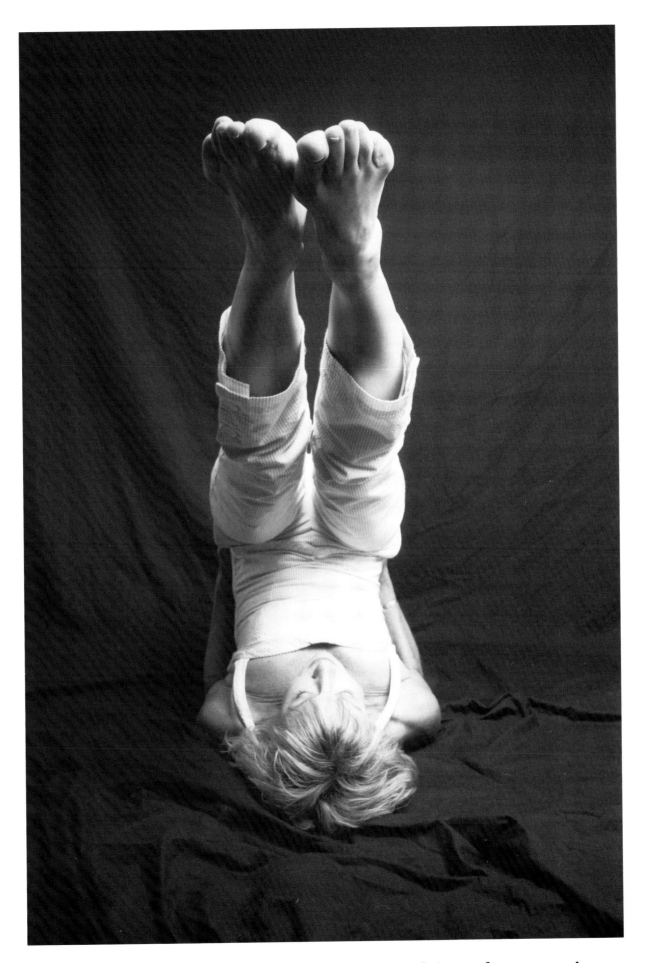

I can always count on Pilates to get back into the groove!

Kaaren Goddess of...Privacy & traveling

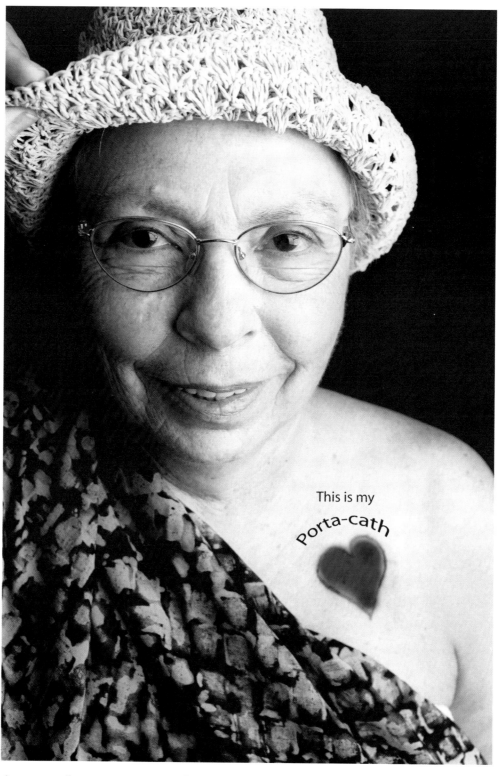

This is my

Porta-cath

I choose to be private because when people know you have cancer,
they treat you differently... I don't like that!

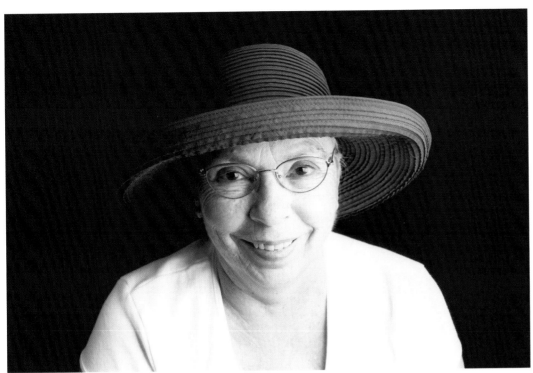

I am 61 years old and was diagnosed with breast cancer in 1984. I had a right side mastectomy without reconstruction. Almost ten years later, the cancer was found in my bones, but this did not hurt. Then the cancer was found in my lungs and liver. I am getting chemotherapy for this.

Nobody has said, "Okay, you are going to die." So, I continue to live my life and travel, especially to Mexico. On second thought, even if someone were to tell me I was going to die tomorrow, I'd pack my bags and run away. **I am alive now!**

Sometimes you feel good, but then you see the results of a scan that is abnormal and you think to yourself--- "That can't be me?!"

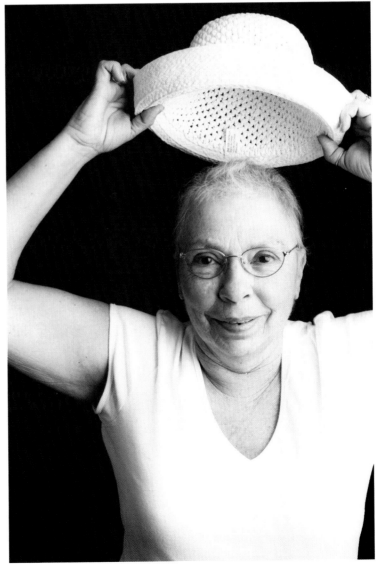

127

Courtney!

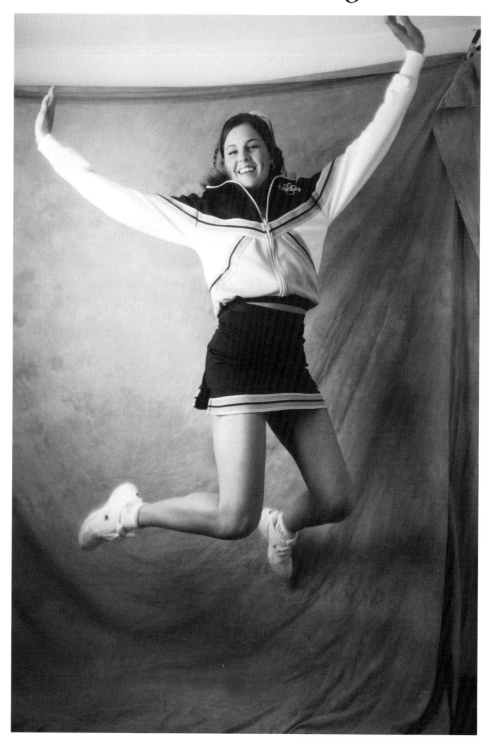

Goddess of... Spunk & Cheerleading

I am 16 years old and have ALL (Acute Lymphocetic Leukemia). I am 5'10" and a cheerleader for my high school: The Buena High Bulldogs. I was diagnosed when I was 14 years old on. One week before, I was making pancakes with my friend when she noticed that my hands were shaking. We started laughing, we realized later that the doctors think I was having a seizure.

In the 9th grade, during cheerleading practice after school, I started to not feel well. I thought, "I have to go to practice!" My mom picked me up early and said, "You look dead!" My lips were white and I was very pale. When I got home, I had a seizure. I fell onto the floor. I bent the window blinds on my way down. My mom took me to the doctor, and I had a temperature of 104.0 degrees and could see my heart beating in my chest when I was lying down. My throat hurt so badly.

Three days later I felt much worse and started to lose weight. I had to go see an ear nose and throat doctor. He drew my blood. The laboratory called that night and said, "There might be a mistake." So we went to the hematologist; apparently my blood count was really abnormal. I did not even know what a "hematologist" was. He was the one who took a bone marrow sample. That hurt really bad. I had never cried so hard. He then said, "Good news, it's not cancer." We were excited. I did need two blood transfusions and had to stay in the hospital. My friends visited me, and my mom then returned to pick me up at 5 o'clock.

The hematologist then came into my hospital room and said to my mom, "You are going to UCLA because Courtney has Leukemia." I had to ride there in an ambulance and my mom rode with me. All I knew about cancer was that I could lose my hair.

Thirteen days later I had another bone marrow test in order to find out what kind of Leukemia I had. Chemotherapy started on October 2, 2000. Within three weeks, I lost my hair. My dad set up a hotline with a pre-recorded message for my friends to hear. I stayed on the cheerleading squad too. I was so concerned about the yearbook picture because I had lost my hair. At first my mom put my hair in two pony tails and cut them off, we saved them and she sewed them into a bandana so it would look like my hair was still on my head and was only sticking out in braids. It was cute.

In the hospital I met another girl that was diagnosed with Leukemia at the same time. We were both on steroids and were always craving food. My older sister had a harder time with me being sick. We are closer now.

I went into remission right away. I have to have three years of chemotherapy, it's all part of a protocol. The first year it was every month. The second year it was given every three months and this last year I have to get it every six months.

I am still a kid. For my last birthday (16th) we rented a "Jolly jump" to play in.

I try to make everyone feel better; I am a mood setter.

I have had 19 blood transfusions so far. They did a blood drive at school and dedicated it to me.

I have lots of close friends and we have fun doing make-overs and laughing. I am proud not to be overly concerned about sex. I prefer sleepovers with my best friends. **Everyone at school thinks I am a hero.**

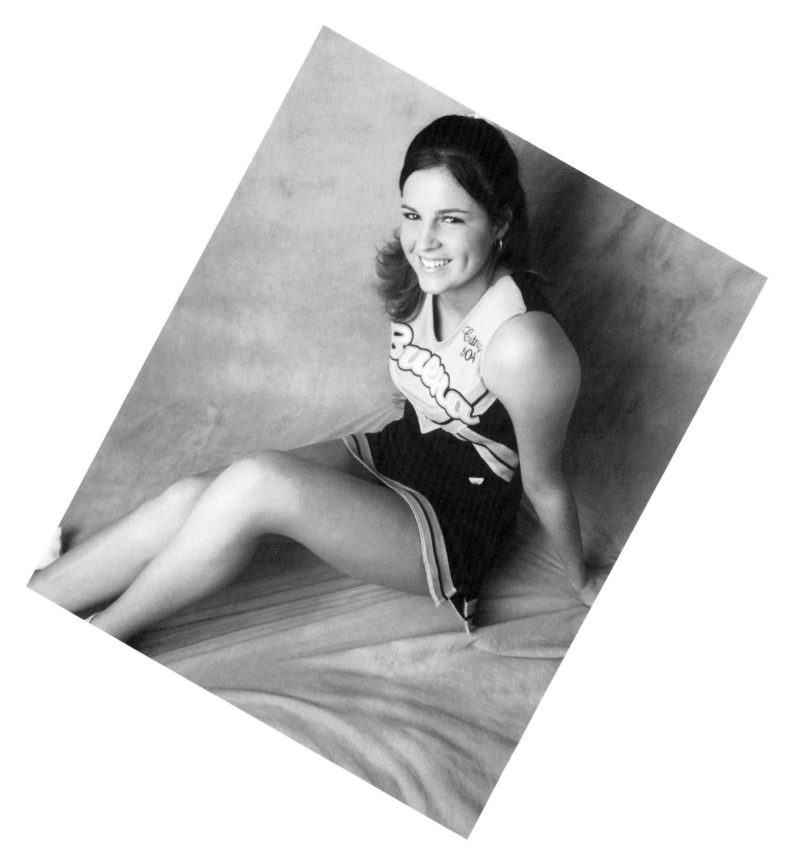

Lance Armstrong said, "Cancer is given to strong people," I can relate to that.

I got to go to "Disneyworld" thanks to the "Make-A-Wish" foundation

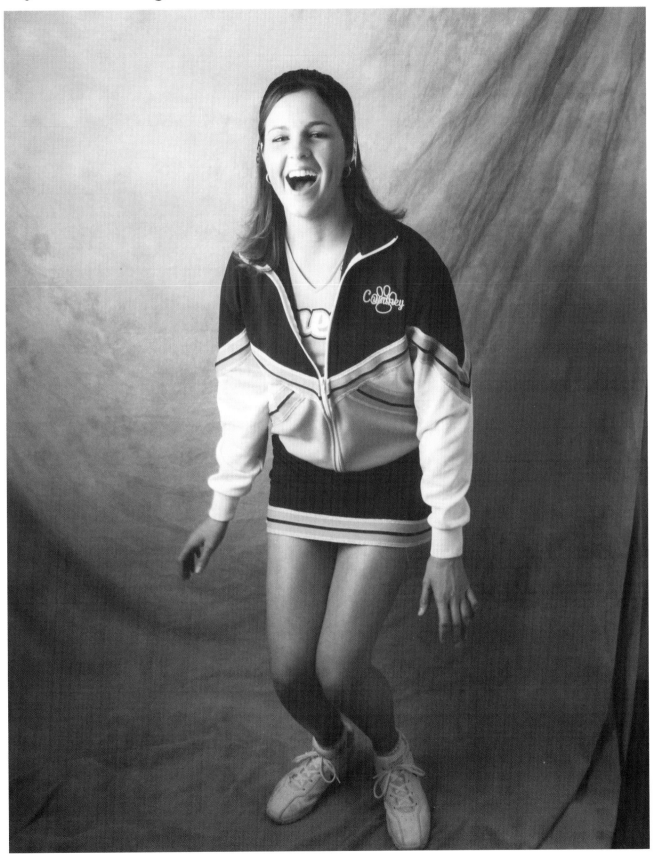

Rachel

Goddess of a long journey, Beating the Odds and Being Bossy!

Rachel's Life Experiences

I have beaten the odds, and even outlived most of my doctors
    I am not into nutrition
I like McDonald's Happy Meals and the toys are great
    The doctor told me I had cancer on Christmas Eve
Cancer is not a gift-- just because it was Christmas time
    I should have died, but instead I'm just a little out of whack
I have had my thyroid removed and have a big scar on my neck
    I started medical school at 35
I don't like doctors, so I decided to become one
    I know 27 different ways to eat Jell-O
Medical school is easy; keeping me alive is the challenge
    After Esophageal cancer, they said I would never speak again...
Ha-Ha, I always speak up
    I am blind in one eye, but I have another one
I am in love—he's truly amazing
    When I am sad I read children's books, they make me laugh
I passed Calculus because I am bossy
       I am tired a lot
     I don't 'get' cancer
I don't like the word "relapse," it sounds so stupid
I have the same friends from high school
      I like to laugh
    Everyday I face infections and new tumors

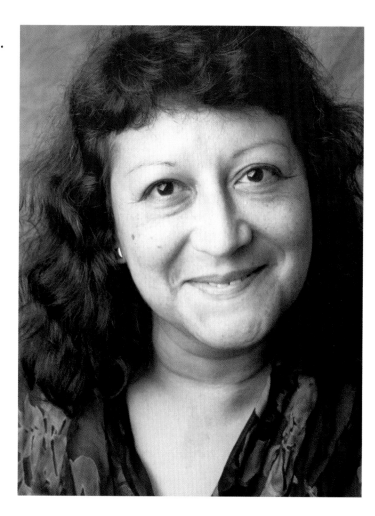

I have outlived most of my doctors!

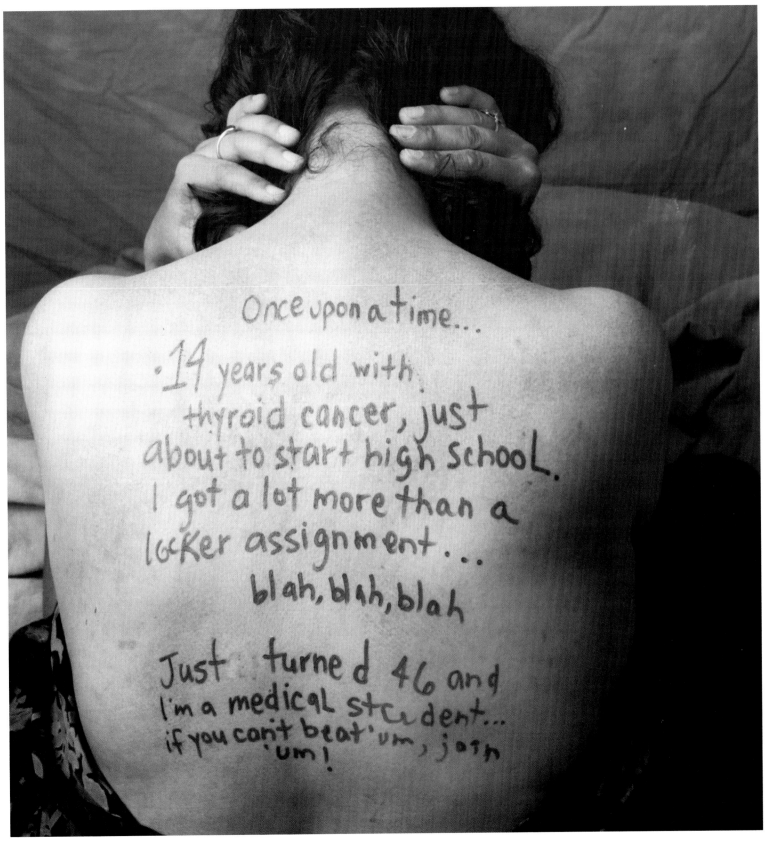

Yesterday I had a huge tumor removed from my mouth.

It will take 10 days to get the pathology report.

All I can do is wait.

I am in *Love* and he helps the time pass.

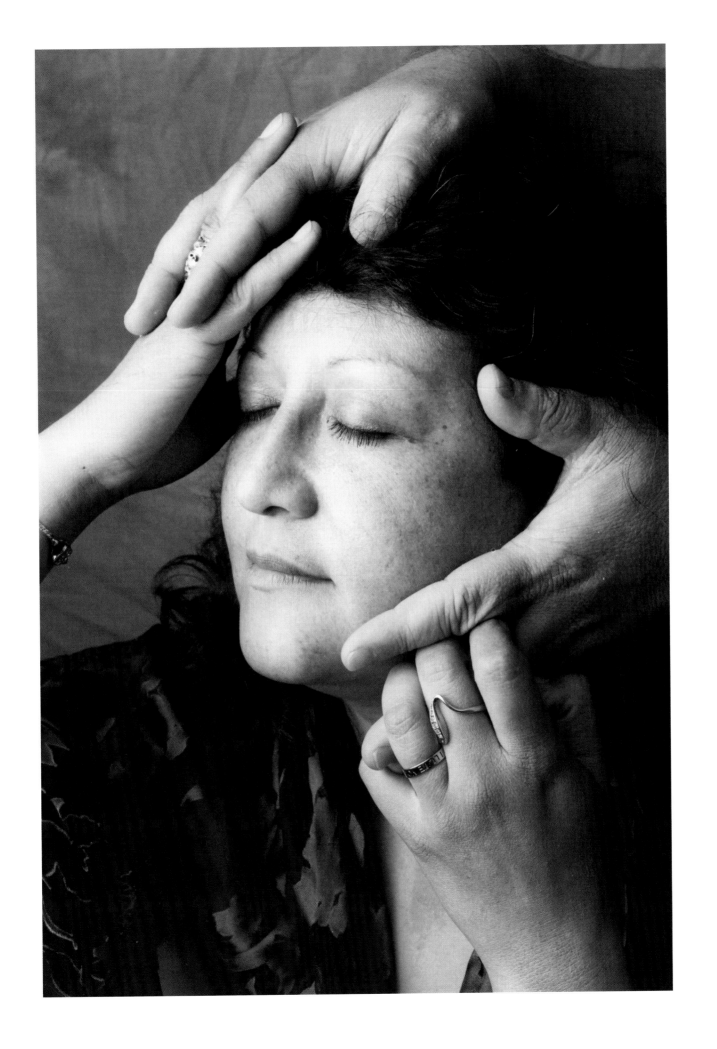

Third time $\longrightarrow$ New encounters

In my years of having cancer, my doctor's office has come a long way. They have made a big turn around. They believe in herbs, reflexology and yoga. This third time, I have witnessed all the advances that medicine has made.

The subject of hair- Well, I don't have much left. I found a wonderful miracle. There is real hair that is woven into my thining hair. It's natural, not humilating, and a great transition for me. Being bald does not freak me out, but thinning hair is just ugly; it's worse being in between.

The cancer came
   back
a third time!

..here I am!

I was four and a half years cancer free, and then the cancer came back. I had a blood test to see if I was a breast cancer gene carrier. Luckily, I am not. I had felt a lump in my neck, but ignored it. My friend Julie encouraged me to see the doctor. He felt my neck on the left side but did not say anything. He did a biopsy and an ultrasound. Seven days later I started chemotherapy. The cancer had returned. I thought, "Three times is a charm?!"

I have been married to my husband Michael for 12 years. He is the one that got me through this third time.

Michael is incredibly supportive. He always made sure that I had the right treatments by the right doctors. We found the best at two hospitals, LA-USC and City of Hope. My doctor is excellent and he is worldly without being a snob.

No matter what, you still need to be your own advocate. You need to know who is treating you and what your treatment options are.

The second time I had a relapse, I thought I would never have chemotherapy again... but here I am. I have too much to live for.

At first I was not strong. I said to my doctor, "I think I need some valium. I am freaking out!" I said this in the room where the other cancer patients were. I got upset in front of them and I cannot believe that I did that.

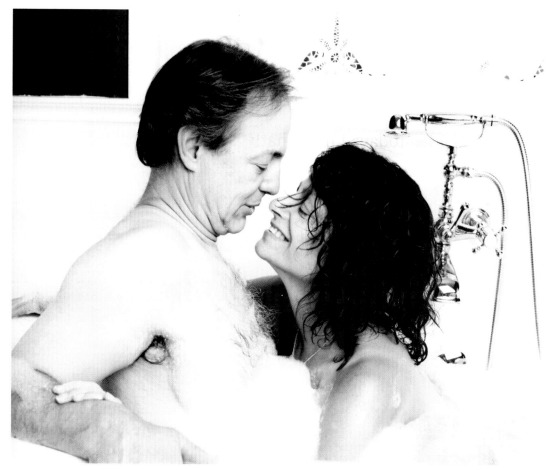

My body did not handle chemotherapy well this time. I got extremely sick and was admitted to the hospital for eight days. My body was toxic and I was in the Intensive Care Unit.

Once again I received a tremendous amount of support. My eight-year-old sons' class made me a gift basket filled with snacks. People brought me bubble bath, chap stick and tranquility music. This was brilliant! I learned to knit and got addicted to crossword puzzles. My mind needed stimulation. I was on a Morphine drip, which caused me to hallucinate. I would knit, but thought I was doing a crossword puzzle. I talked to myself. I was a mess, but it was comical.

People prayed for me. I had been 'NPO,' which meant no food or water. I became anorexic and weighed 80 pounds. My brother came to visit and brought me what we call *Jewish Penicillin*- chicken soup. "Just EAT!" he demanded. The soup stimulated my appetite. Once I started eating, I was able to go home. I was touched and impressed by my brother's nurturing.

The cancer was caught early. You don't hear about someone surviving a third time. Once again, I can value that you need to live for today. I am stubborn. If there is something I consider important, I do it now. I am not waiting. I do not have as much patience as others do. I just want to live. This is good and bad. The good is that I think positive and I am not a downer. The bad is that other people don't always recognize the urgency that I have.

This last round, my husband played the wife, father, friend and everything else. We cried and laughed together. Being sick is not easy, especially with a big household; there is always some kind of family drama.

Michael was there to answer everyone's questions. I can tell him my deepest secrets, the kind that you usually can't say to people. I can always be honest with him. We even talked about my funeral and the songs that he would play. I am an optimistic, but a realist too.

The bone marrow transplants that I had bought me more life. I am lucky that I had a four year remission. The doctors are learning a lot from my illness. They are now further educated on how to treat other people and me with the same disease.

The cure has come a long way. Now there are vaccine studies and genetic studies to find a cure.

I feel good today. I have that!

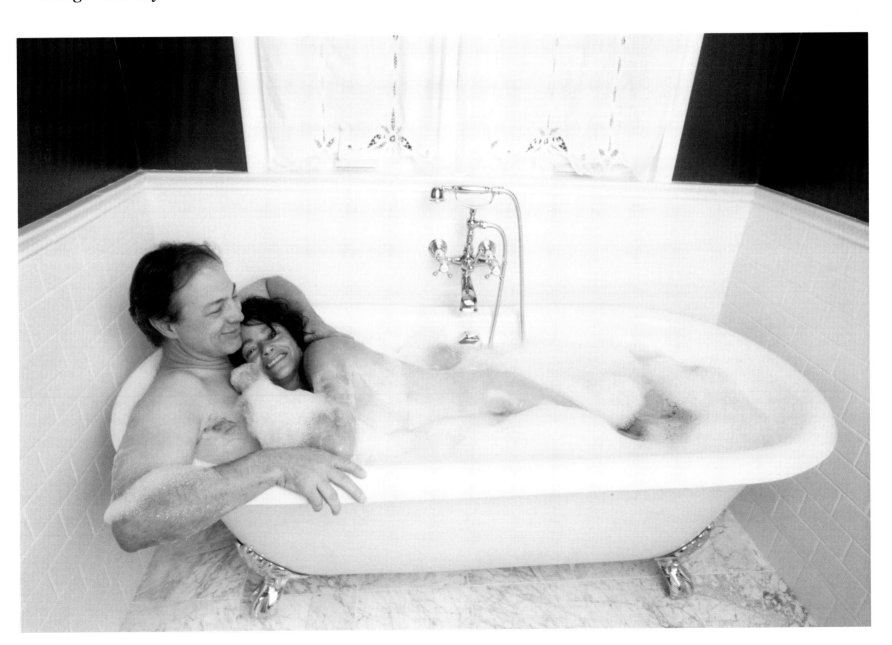

This book is dedicated to...

To our son: Jim met his lymphoma "challenge' with tremendous grace and strength. He continually provided us with hope when we should have been the providers. We are indeed proud of Jim and happy that we could be with him through much of his treatment. We make this dedication with a great deal of love. Mama Pajama and Padre'

My grandmother's strength and sacrifice gave my mom her strength to be a survivor, through me their strength has been given to my daughter. Evvi Sutherland

I wish to dedicate a short memory for beloved parents--Adolfe and Emilie Hahn (Brager) who brought me up to love and enjoy life. They never had a change to se me get married, hold their grandchildren and great grandchildren. Their life was cut short by dying in a concentration camp, Aushwitz in 1944. Their memory lives on through me, my children and my family.
Irma Rosenberg   OMI

Jack Gallagher...To Action Jackson, I miss your wisdom. Thanks for coming into my life! Love, Toot

Jerry Standiford...A great man, friend, father and lover. God Bless him! Flo Isbell

Elsie Irene Hillman.... In loving memory, you were an awesome inspiration and wonderful role model as mother, daughter, wife, nurse, neighbor and friend. Thank you for all the lessons in loves! Your grateful daughter Karen

To my sister and brother, Yale Ezratty & Vivian Ezratty.... Love, Your sister Linda Rosenberg

Dorothea Daugherty, Robert Dean Daugherty & Carol Elson....
They have each lost their battle with cancer, but fought it to their limits with dignity & grace.   Bronwyn Ensor

My parents..Bill & Elizabeth Allen, both survivors of cancer.   My dear friend Reenie Holly who unfortunately is no longer here but her spirit certainly is.   Melinda Wellman

To my mom Julie Glickman! Love, your son David Glickman

My mom and daughter Brie...To two of the most important women in my life. I love you, Clancy

To Mrs. M...because the sun rises when you get up in the morning. Thank you for your love and wisdom. Love, Kelly Seitner

To all the women that have lost their lives to cancer.   You are amazing! Love, Judy Bennis

To my dad, Your strength continues to amaze me. I love you. Melinda Palmer

To my Aunt Mary Francis Shannon...a breast cancer survivor! Love, Suzan Rogers

My mom...Norma Lytle who died of cancer in 2001. Love, Larry Lytle

To Cousin Margaret Edith Trussell...better known to us as Mees. She was a strong independent woman. She would do anything for you without compromising her own beliefs and somehow was able to do just about everything she wanted to do. She was a college professor and always a teacher, a writer and published her own books. She fought her cancer her way and kept up the good fight even when faced with Parkinsons Disease. She loved dogs and always had one by her side (mostly yellow labs). We all admired her. With much love, John and Jan Elmore

For Judee M. Ryan - My little sister-a hero to me in so many ways. Know that I am always there. Love, Sisa

To my mother, Diane, who is the epidemy of beauty, strength and selflessness. Love, Melissa

Bill was an inspiration to everyone he touched. He still inspires me, and he's been gone more than six years now.
He had a way of making everyone feel special – he taught me that each of us IS special, unique, capable of good, of fun.
Bill taught me to love life. To notice the many beautiful colors of life. And to be dignified and appreciative when leaving it.
Each day I strive to walk straight and confident and tall like he did, to be a wonderful and loving parent, spouse, and friend.
To be just and fear not - to trust my inner voice. I am a better person thanks to Bill. I cherish each memory and am grateful
for every second I was privileged to share with this special human. I will never AGAIN meet anyone like him.
What a lucky woman I am to have been loved by Bill Keene. Bill, I'll see you upstairs someday –
maybe there you can really teach me to surf, Love Margalit

To my treasured friend Gayle...who will always be my role model. Thanks to her, I now believe we can continue to celebrate life
in the midst of chaos and suffering. Julie Hoffman

To my husband Frank and 3 daughters...Lori, Marci and Melanie. Thank you for your courage to sit with my tears. Linda Montoya

George A. Gerbenskey 1933-2002...My dad fought hard to the end when the cancer went to his liver.
He was a mere 85 pounds when we lost him. He will always be our hearts. Jean Myers

John & Nancy McCarthy...Brother and sister who will live with us forever. Jean Myers

To Grandpa, Aunt Nancy, and Uncle John: Don't cry because it's over Smile because it happened. Love, Cassidy

To my precious children, Hanna, Pierre and Colin. Love, Mommy (Edna Dangiapo)

To David Peltz--A husband, father, grand-father & mentor to many. You are missed by all whose lives you touched.
Eight years was not enough time to have with you. A soulmate comes only once in alifetime. I miss my best friend.
I will meet you at rainbow bridge. Love, Cindy P.S. When we had to have Mr. B (our cat) put down, the vets office sent us
this beautiful card telling the story of rainbow bridge. It is where all pets who pass on go to wait for there masters.
The grass is green and the hills are full of flowers that never die. There is no more pain for anyone who stays there.
Your dad and Iagreed that when he or I passed, we would wait for each other with Mr. B at the bridge.
I know he is there waiting.

To Hortencia--- YOU ROCK! Love Amy DeSario

I am so thankful to be surrounded by guardian angels here on earth and in heaven. Every day I know that I am loved.
They cushion the fall when they can and pick me up when I fall. I am the luckiest person in the world! Joy Clausen

To Annie Bates, Love Dee Johnston

The survivors in this book remind me of my own personal hero, Jim Hoag. My uncle Jim was wheelchair-bound from
Multiple Sclerosis when I was a young girl. Despite his disability, he was my "most fun" relative and our favorite babysitter.
He never lost his sense of adventure or his remarkable wit and charm, even in his last days.
He continues to be an inspiration to all who knew him. Holly Carlisle

To my mother Marlene - strong in spirit, gentle in heart. To the world you might be one person, but to me, you are the world.
Love Tina Coates

THANK YOU!
All these wonderful people helped with the publication of this book....

Sandi & Randy Anderson, Jason & Sharon Anderson, Chrispin Andes, Paulo Andes, Aprhodites, Ana Capa Bakery
Fred & Judy Bysshe, Win & Melissa Banning, Ruth & James Bullock, Holly, Troy & Kate Barkley,
Brian & Andrea @ Aptos Creek Vineyard, Juliet Brown, Markalaka & Jannaramma Borgers,
Chris & Tim Brzycki, Tom & Mary Barlett, Black light Band, Lisa & Jim Buerle, Richard & Betsy Burns,
Gayle & Michael Brinkenhoff, Dari Cohn, Judy Bennis, Linda & Mark Barker, Mia @ Cara Mia,
Bob & Manette Cooper, Jen Chatiner & Rachel Livingston, Kaye Kaye Chase, Holly Carlisle, Joy Clausen,
Friends @ C & R Repographics, Mandy & Sergio Cannone, Amy Crittenden & Lorelle Dawes, Jill Davis,
Everyone @ Celebs salon, Dayna @ Babycakes, Sharon Breese, Danny Cangemi, Tina Coates,
Dr. Coleen Copelan & Dr. Ron Thurston, Clare Davey & James O'Kelly, Roger & Blance Dykehouse,
Sharon & Erik Dahl, Baby Jen & Sergio, Dayna @ Babycakes, Devin & Amy DeSario, Edna Dangiapo,
John & Jayme Dwyer, Friends @ Danny's Deli, Anne & Bill Daley,
Master James Evans & Premier Martial Arts Family, Bronwyn & Gary Ensor,
Jan & John Elmore,Sonny & Clarice Feinberg, Gloria Forgea, Sandy @ Fruition, Kirk & Jennifer Flittie,
Jill & Marc Fiorvanti, Joe Glickman, David Glickman & Dario Diaz, Daniel & Hahn Garcia,
Victoria & Dan Graham, The Goddesses, Gerald & Barbara Gustave, Dave & Katie Ganzer,
Nathalie & Rudy Gonzales, Marques Guy, Ruth & Rich Hoag, Natalie Hilley, Heidi @ Comforts,
Dr Ian Hollsworth, Stace & Dan Hicks, Nate & Teri Hunt, Julie & Rob Hoffman,
Danine & Michael Holbert @ Victoria Pub, Natalie Hilley, Karen Hillman-Castelan, Donna & Joe Heany,
Flo Henderson, Bill & Cindy Hendricks, All the staff @ The Image Source, Amy Jones & Dina Pielaet
John @ Calico Stained Glass, Dee Johnston, Pat Kim, Deke Klatt, Dana & Pat Kearney,
Flo Isbell & Bob VanWyngarden, Don & Kitty Lockwood, John & Bridget Lee, Nicole Luboff,
Lisa Lambright & James Sherman, Cindy Lee, Derek Lisoski, Phyllis & Bob Knorr, Julie Miller, Luke Matjas
Dionne Myers & Scott Vett, Jean & Ken Myers, Katherine McGuire, Jason Mukerjee & Jessica Frey, Jaqi Malone,
Thad Matuszesju & Gargi Dasguptua, Linda & Lori Montoya, Sharon Manisco, Joy & Tom Nairne,
Natalie @ Natalie's Fine Threads, Roberta & Harry Nelson, Kiley Olivier, Gloria & Doug Otten,
Cindy Peltz & Rebecca & Olivia, Charles & Yvette Pierson, Lesley Paarmann, Johanna Pimental,
Abra & David Paudler, Melinda Palmer, Tina @ Pet Barn, Diane Patton, Adam Peltz & Cassidy McCarthy,
Suzan & Charlie Rogers, Natalie Rimmele, Linda Byrne & Luke McAuliffe, Larry Lytle,
Linda & Stanley Rosenberg, Irma Rosenberg, Jonathan & Michelle Rosenberg, Jeff & Nicole Raven,
Lyn & Jeff Rauls, Evelyn & Jim Sutherland, Steven & Kimber Sax, Gregory Schuh,
Shannon @ Ladybug & Caterpillar, Linda & Bud Sloan, Ron Sinton, Kelly & Joe Seither,
Steve & Jeannine Serbanich, Sara Smelt, Nancy & Kenny Sutherland, Friends @ The Side Car Resturant,
Kyle & Tammy Swanson, Suzanne Saw, Joyce & Pat Sheehan, Everyone @ Shamsi's Deli, Avery & Tracy Stewart,
Bonnie Sessions, Tammy & Jeff Robinson, Stuart Tower, John & Maria Tregaskiss, Giovanni Tramba @ Table 13,
Gail, Tom, Nick & Lindsay Trumble, Margalit & Lee Tocher, Anne & Syed Salahuddin, Michele & Dave Rozo
Violet @ Violets Rubber Stamp Inn, Marnie Volpe, Lou Valdez, Rob Webber, Deborah Wicken,
Melinda & Ken Wellman, Dr Robert & Dr Wendy WarWar, Jan & Joe Wurts,
Jen Wood, Shirley Westover, Donna Wood, Julie Vanoni, Ventura Veterinary Medical & Surgical Group,
The All Girl band that played at my benefit: Amy, Sheila, Linda, Vicki & Nancy

Thank You...

Jim, **my love** and **my hero**. Thank you for never giving up!!!

My mom Evvi and Ladder-Dad Jim: Thank you for giving us strength

My daddy-dumeature: Thank you for your conviction & watching over us

My brother Adam... Thank you for your friendship & for the awesome front cover design

Thank you Omi-you are absolutely amazing

Jim's parents Anne & Bill Daley: Thank you for holding our hands and hearts through out--from the begining

Sammy Sealion, Mailie Bean and Moon Ri: Thank you for your unconditional puppy love

To Holly-Walter: "The road to a friends house is never long." Thank you!

Cindy, Becca & Olivia; family by marriage, connected by love

Collen Copelan: Thank you for keeping us sane

Dr Kelley & Staff: Thank you for saving Jim's life

CHOP & Rituxan: Thank you to all the scientists who discovered these medications

Bill Hendricks: Thank you for pushing me to be the best photographer I can be

Najja Foluke: Thank you for being my friend from miles and through the years

Chris Cryer: Thank you for all the professional English knowledge you gave so kindly

David Duperre: Thank you for being the only literary agent to believe in this project

To the friends who shaved their heads to support Jim: Rob Webber, Scott Vett, Greg Schuh, Dr. Tom Richards, Adam Peltz and Kyle Swanson. Thank you Erik Rinde for your razor!

The Cancer Center of Ventura County: Thank you for the support groups and a place to feel normal

Thank you to all the Goddesses in this book! Thank you for your willingness to share your stories and glory

Thank you to my wonderful girlfriends: Abra, Amy, Baby Jen, Dionne, Gail, Gloria, Jill, Jeannine, Kiley, Natalie & Sara! I love you

Thank you, Hello Kitty & Tori Amos my two "secret" friends!

Thank you Dina for all your time, patience and guidance. You rock!
Thank you Jeff @ colorworks printing (in Ventura, California) for printing my dream.

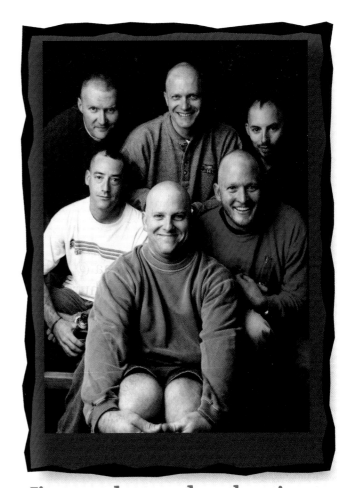

Jim...my love and my hero!
When Jim lost his hair from Chemotherapy, my brother and several friends shaved their heads to support him.

This book comes from my heart and all the cells in my body. The inspiration I received from the Goddesses in the book, carried me through the entire production of this project.

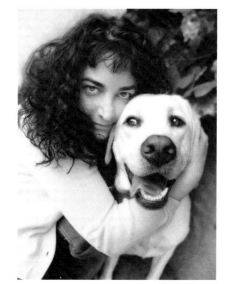

Moon Ri Polar bear

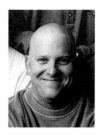

*"Here's to the crazy ones,
the misfits,
the rebels,
the troublemakers,
the round pegs in the square holes,
the ones who see things differently.
They're not fond of rules,
and they have no respect for the status quo.
You can quote them
disagree with them, glorify or vilify them...
about the only thing you can't do is ignore them,
because they change things,
they push the human race forward.
And while some may see them as the crazy ones,
we see genius,
because the people who
are crazy enough to think they can change the world
are the ones who do."*

Poem from The Apple Macintosh Computer Ad

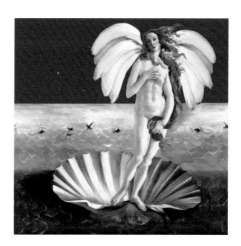

Please visit: Goddessbook.com